Effective Case Records for Substance Related Disorders

Sherry S. Kimbrough

Landon L. Kimbrough

Southworth Press

PORT TOWNSEND · WASHINGTON

Southworth Press
4663 Mason Street
Port Townsend, Washington 98368
www.lanstat.com

Book Layout ©2013 BookDesignTemplates.com

Ordering Information:
Quantity sales. Special discounts are available on quantity purchases by corporations, associations, and others. For details, contact the "Sales Department" at the address above.

Effective Case Records for Substance Related Disorders / Sherry Kimbrough & Landon Kimbrough —1st ed.
ISBN 978-0-578-14908-0

Contents

This book is lovingly dedicated to Gerry Coughlin who was a co-author of our previous books and urged us to write another.
She is a co-author in spirit.
Gerry began her career in the substance abuse disorder field in 1974. The creator and facilitator of hundreds of continuing education experiences, she attributed her love of teaching to "being a ham." Her mentor, Father James Royce, invited her to help develop the first case-management class for academic credit. She went on to profoundly affect the treatment of alcoholics and drug addicts with her teaching and supervision and received a number of awards for her efforts.

Gerry passed away in December of 2013. She is missed intensely by her friends and colleagues in the field. She was an original.

Introduction

Since our first edition of Patient Records and Addiction Treatment in 1996, the substance abuse disorder treatment field continues to undergo changes that affect the contents of this book. In an effort to include information that assists students and practitioners to use best practices, we have substantially revised and retitled this book.

This book was developed originally because in teaching the case management course and similar courses at colleges and universities for several years, the authors had not found a suitable text to use as a guide. After attempting to provide this level of information through lectures and many handouts, we felt that the information would be easier to assimilate if organized into book form.

Our format integrates current information and research, principles of sound clinical practice and practical experience. Our intention is to outline the procedures and rationale of case management and clinical documentation to give readers some background as well as information regarding current practice.

In addition to our history as instructors and workshop leaders, we have provided direct services to patients and furnished clinical supervision for substance abuse disorder treatment providers. Currently most of our work falls into the consulting arena where we are asked to provide guidance regarding agency operations and quality improvement. Two primary tenets that guide our work and this book are:

- Better clinical records equal better treatment outcomes.
- Good record keeping facilitates an effective treatment team approach.

A variety of factors has seemingly increased the paperwork load on substance abuse disorder counselors. Many organizations now use clinical record software or a combination of electronic and paper records. Using an electronic medical record (EMR) has some very real advantages over paper records, such as reducing duplication of effort. It is important to understand that using an EMR, while supporting timely and consistent recordkeeping, should not be a shortcut resulting in sloppy records. Attention to detail is just as crucial to good recordkeeping when using an electronic record. Templates for various tasks can be a tangible time saver and help with consistency but are not a substitute for clinical judgment.

Our goal for this book is to give our readers a good grounding in the practical reasons and methods concerning case records, as well as some tips to streamline the process. The more accomplished a clinician becomes in recordkeeping, the more time they have available to spend with the individuals they serve.

This model is based primarily on the records requirements for international accreditation and Washington State, which is one of the states that mandates a number of specific record elements. We believe that this model will portray the essential elements of a good recordkeeping system, and good recordkeeping practice, no matter where an organization is located.

It is our hope that you find this book helpful to your current practice, whether you are a beginner or an experienced clinician.

CHAPTER 1

Levels of Care and Recordkeeping

"The horror of that moment," the King went on, "I shall never never forget!" "You will, though," the Queen said, "if you don't make a memorandum of it."

— Lewis Carroll

Substance related disorder treatment includes a variety of types of care and services. Depending on the type and duration of service, records can vary considerably from organization to organization. This book will identify some of the common types of treatment included under the rubrics "addiction," or "substance abuse" or "chemical dependency" treatment and their requisite case records. Specialty treatment, particularly that which involves medical interventions and medication can be more complicated, but the rules and standards articulated in this book are applicable.

Initial Contact

Looking at substance related disorder treatment from an initial viewpoint, the first point of contact may be a call center or a screener such as the receptionist on a telephone at a treatment center. This contact is vitally important when it comes to the person's willingness to continue with the process to begin treatment. Properly trained staff will know what information to gather and how to obtain the essential data to assist the person. The staff person must be cognizant that they are assisting the individual on the first action to begin their recovery journey, as well as providing encouraging and helpful knowledge. The goal is to begin the development of a partnership, to get the potential patient person seeking help engaged. This also helps to reduce resistance and the caller is more likely to follow through. Announcing that the facility is full can be a deal-breaker. Sometimes an invitation to come to visit the facility can be effective. At that time a future admission date can be discussed.

Screening

A screening form is often the first component of a treatment case file. It will generally include the presenting problem – why the person made the contact – and basic information about the individual. Documentation of the individual's eligibility for treatment, including funding options and whether or not the organization can provide the services needed are also essential. In the case of a significant other or a referent making the call, obtaining their information as well as a means to contact them is very important.

Screening forms should show the disposition of the call: what happened and whether the person was referred on elsewhere, made an appointment or simply broke off contact. Follow up on referrals is often tracked on this form also. In a best practice environment, the information on the form, such as where the individual came from or heard about the center, what happened next, and a follow-up contact (as appropriate) is tracked and the results are analyzed by management for planning and service adjustments.

Sometimes the first form used to begin the file is a referral from another organization (see figure 1). If this information is received prior to the first contact with the individual, a call to set up an appointment may be necessary and helpful. The initiating referral should include a release of information to allow communication with the prospective patient and the referring agency. Generally the referral information is accompanied by a release of information (see Chapter 3) and any questions about the information should be clarified by the receiving agency.

Numerous studies have shown that a handwritten card or letter or a telephone call as a follow-up to an initial visit drastically increase the return by a prospective patient. Likewise, being able to see a person immediately upon their contact, however briefly, rather than assigning a later appointment can reduce attrition.[1]

Screening Instruments

Once the individual has arrived at the treatment location, a number of other assessment forms should be completed. If screening or assessment tools are used they should be uniformly administered, field recognized and validated instruments. Any personnel using the tools instruments should be trained prior to administering them and this training documented. Should questions arise in the future regarding scores or decisions made based on these scores, it's important to have this backup. Remember, test scores are only a tool, not a diagnosis!

Assessment

Contingent on the condition of the patient individual seeking help and the type of treatment, the first visit may be a full assessment or just a brief evaluation to determine the urgent needs, often called a triage assessment or risk assessment. A triage assessment will focus on the current physical needs of the person: risk of withdrawal and/or complicating illnesses of an urgent nature. A crisis assessment may be conducted as well, documenting, if found: suicide risk or danger to self or others. Contingent Depending on the services offered by the organization, the person's status in the area of basic needs such as food or shelter may also be assessed. Triage assessment is different from an extended screening in that only limited areas are assessed and minimal plans made; a person may be referred directly to a physician for a history and physical to obtain medication or for the resolution of an emergent life issue, such as domestic violence or no place to sleep for the night. In all cases, the specific assessment process should be tailored to the age, language capabilities and physical condition of the person being assessed. Documentation that this customization look at urgent individual needs has taken place is important to include in the assessment summary we will discuss later. It is important to include these areas of assessment in the assessment summary, which we will discuss later.

Screening, Brief Intervention, and Referral to Treatment (SBIRT)

The Substance Abuse and Mental Health Service Administration (SAMHSA) began an initiative several years ago to integrate a brief assessment into primary health care and other community settings. SBIRT is a public health approach to the delivery of early intervention and treatment services for people with substance use disorders and those at risk of developing these disorders. Many different types of community settings provide opportunities for early intervention with at-risk substance users before more severe consequences occur. SBIRT is a comprehensive, integrated, public health approach to the delivery of early intervention and treatment services for persons with substance use disorders, as well as those who are at risk of developing these disorders. Primary care centers, hospital emergency rooms, trauma centers, and other community settings provide opportunities for early intervention with at-risk substance users before more severe consequences occur. Individuals are referred to the treatment site after their screening and intervention.

First Visit

Depending on the desires and needs of the person, the first contact may focus on the presenting concern and not on collecting a substantial amount of history. It is important to create a partnership with the person at this stage and At this stage it is vital to show showing them that you are interested in their concerns is vital in order to create a partnership with the person. Many persons individuals seen in substance related treatment facilities are in need of the level of screening described in triage, but once any emergent issues are either resolved or deferred, the contact will proceed to a full psychosocial assessment.

If conducted, this full assessment includes an in depth look at a variety of many life areas: current and past health, psychological and relationship status, legal involvement, if any, and employment and living situations. The information from this assessment should result in an assessment summary which includes the desires of the patient, the evaluation of the clinician and the likely first steps to reach the patient's goals. An assessment and summary of this type is essential to any form of service planning.

Service Planning

Contingent on the level of care, the service plan will vary in scope from a routine focus on current acute medical issues, such as withdrawal, to longer term and perhaps more intransigent difficulties. In the chapter on service planning we will focus on the planning process itself. No matter the level of care, a plan must be developed. In the case of a medical facility or opioid substitution service, the initial plan may take the form of a protocol, or standard service plan, based on doctor's orders. The service planning process must be documented, and progress noted. Elements of the service process can be found in figure 1 (below). The plan and notes of progress are the heart of the patient record and keep track of the path of the individual through service. The master service plan will likely itemize a number of issues, and each issue assigned a number. Progress is noted on both the plan itself and in notes that may be filed away from the plan in the case record. When the progress notes are on a separate form, they should be designated as relating to a specific service plan.

Primary Record Elements of the Service Process

1. Patient makes first contact:
   a. Screening forms completed either over the phone by phone or in person
   b. Appointment or referral
2. Assessment takes place:
   a. Information gathering
   b. Diagnosis
   c. Summary
   d. Referral or placement
3. Patient enters service:
   a. Service plan
   b. Progress notes

   c. Case reviews
   d. Record reviews
4. Patient transitions:
   a. Transition plan
   b. Discharge summary

Fig. 1

Documenting Services and Progress

Subject to the level of care and goals of service, the file may contain a large variety of tests and test results, patient generated material, legal papers, and mandated forms for signature. Each level of care should have available for reference a list of required forms and formats for their particular needs. Developing a sample "mock" file containing all required paperwork can be quite helpful, especially to a new clinician. For an EMR, a protocol should be developed.

Ongoing service progress may be documented in a variety of ways. A note for an educational session should contain, at a minimum, the title of the curriculum being presented. If the service session is a daily event, or happens several times a day, a sign in sheet for each patient that is filled out and put in the file when completed may be the best method. Sign-in sheets with patient feedback can be used for group in a less intensive level of care, including a place for the clinician's comments on participation. Different methods for documenting service may be used, as long as the method clearly identifies whom the note is regarding and by whom it is being written. Progress notes should always include the date, duration, and outcome or type of event, or comment on progress.

Transition and Discharge

Prior to discharge from any level of care, evidence of transition planning should appear in the record. Transition is defined as the patient's individual's movement from a more intensive to a less intensive level of care. An transition example is stepping down from residential service to outpatient service. A transition plan should include items identified in service planning that are unresolved, as well as what support is available in the community.

Creating a formal transition plan (sometimes called an aftercare plan) can be very helpful for an individual who will be relying less on clinical services. Statements about goals and progress can be helpful, as well as information about resources to deal with problems that may arise. Examples are information about self-help, continuing medications and/or important phone numbers.

A discharge summary should be prepared for any patient who leaves a level of care, regardless of their reason for leaving. The summary clearly states what the presenting issues were and what progress has been made at the time of discharge. A discharge summary is prepared whether or not the individual completed service satisfactorily. Unlike the transition plan, the discharge summary is a clinical document, prepared for the information of another clinician who may be admitting the patient to their service setting or who may reopen the patient file at a later date. Information about anticipated or completed follow-up contacts could be included here.

Chapter Review

· Why is the initial contact so important?

· What factors are taken into account in the decision to do a triage or full assessment?

· Name four elements of a patient record and their use in patient are.

Notes

[1] BIEN, T. H., MILLER, W. R. and TONIGAN, J. S. (1993), Brief interventions for alcohol problems: a review. Addiction, 88: 315–336

CHAPTER 2

Best Practices for Case Records

"Write while the heat is in you. The writer who postpones the recording of his thoughts uses an iron which has cooled to burn a hole with. He cannot inflame the minds of his audience."

— Henry David Thoreau

A well managed organization uses a comprehensive clinical record system governed by recognized principles of health record management. While the primary legal responsibility for case records rests with the administrator, this duty is generally delegated to the clinical person in charge, often known as the Clinical Supervisor.

Case records should be organized, complete, clear and current. Reasonable protection from damage caused by fire, flood or other hazards is expected for both active current and inactive records. Organizations using EMR must ensure that safety, security and backup procedures are in place. These include, in part, screen savers, log-ins for staff members, routine backup procedures with off-site storage of backup media and ways to verify media. Any disclosures of information taking place electronically must be encrypted.

Security and Confidentiality of Records

Access to records is limited to staff members who have a need to access the records, such as appropriate clinical and administrative staff members. This is accomplished by log-in permissions for EMR and securing paper records in either locked file cabinets or locked rooms. While keeping records secure is certainly an ethical principle, in the case of alcohol and drug service records, it is also a legal one, as defined in 42CFR, Part 2. Case records should be controlled from a central location to ensure consistency and confidentiality.

Case Record System

Case records are usually ordered alphabetically or by an assigned number, and often by program in a multi program organization. Individuals are frequently assigned a unique number upon admission, consisting, for example, of the first four letters of the individual's last name and the last four digits of their social security number. This device is used for a variety of reasons. In some cases, as in a very large agency, county or state system, it is used to confirm the identity of a particular individual. It may also be employed in research or among organization personnel to designate individuals without using their names and thereby breaking confidentiality. If a paper case file is used, a record of all individuals' full names and identifiers might be computerized as a cross reference.

Today, most organizations are using a completely computerized system. This computerized record or records system should be maintained with confidentiality in mind. This includes computers that contain billing information as well as clinical information. Passwords should be known to select administrative staff and kept in a secure location.

Case Record Contents

The service provider should maintain a clinical records system comprised of clearly identifiable records for each modality of treatment. Forms that provide all the required record information should be readily available, either in paper or electronic media. Staff members must be fully oriented to the clinical record system prior to beginning individual care and the agency must have a system to ensure this. Good record keeping facilitates good treatment. Figure 2 shows how information gathering and the resulting documentation provide structure for the treatment process.

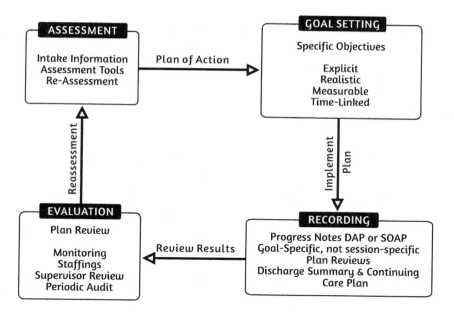

Fig. 2

Minimum Case Records Content

- Full name
- Home address
- Telephone number
- Date of birth
- Individual record number (as appropriate)
- Emergency contact and/or next of kin
- Admission date
- Discharge date
- Referral source
- Current status

Important Items That Should Be Included, As Necessary, in Case Records

- Authentication record
- Authorization to release information
- Consent to service
- Correspondence - a note referencing each correspondence should also be in the progress notes.
- Discharge summary
- Evidence of the direct involvement of individuals in service planning
- Evidence of reviews, both clinical and quality assurance
- Financial arrangements
- Follow-up information
- Intake/Assessment form
- Medical reports
- Progress notes
- Records of family conferences
- Referrals
- Team conferences/Continued service reviews

· Individual Service Plans
· Transition plans and referrals

Authentication

Case record content is completed and authenticated with the signature (full name and title) of the person providing the observation, evaluation, or service. An EMR that restricts access or automatically identifies the person entering the data meets this requirement.

In paper records or logs, it was previously best practice to assure that all entries be made in black ink. Current practice suggests that blue may be better to assist in differentiating an original from a copy. Additionally, supervisors or individuals doing quality review may make notations in another color. The organization should have a policy regarding records that clearly states what color ink is to be used in what circumstances.

Using consistent time frames and forms for entries is vital to good clinical practice. A policy and procedure should exist that includes the amount of time allowed to make an entry: within one business day of the service delivery or event, for example,. The format in which entries will be made should also be included.

Record Retention and Storage

Case records are retained for a minimum time period after the date of the last entry in the record. This time period may range from five to ten years after the discharge or transfer of the individual. The retention time varies dependent on the state and federal regulations and funding sources contractual requirements. After the prerequisite time interval the records may be destroyed in a manner that maintains the confidentiality of the record.

If electronic software is being used for case files, be sure to consult your software provider about how to effectively erase files.

Before you sell, donate, or recycle your old computer, beware, as you may be handing personal information to strangers. Simply restoring the operating system to factory settings does not delete all data and neither does formatting the hard drive before reinstalling the OS. To really wipe a drive clean, you will need to run secure-erase software.[1]

As discussed previously, the organization should have a secure storage system that protects active and inactive records from inadvertent damage during storage. In the event that the organization closes permanently, arrangements need to be made for the continued management of case records until the pre-destruction obligatory time interval has elapsed. Some organizations have a policy that states that any destruction of records is stopped if a legal action is pending toward the organization. This is to insure that any records pertinent to an action will be retained.

Progress Notes

From the first moment of individual contact, the clinician becomes responsible and accountable to the individual, the community, the profession, the payer, co-workers, and a legal system that protects the rights of each individual. Any and all individual contacts, whether face to face, by phone or in a group should be documented. In addition, any consultation or referral done on behalf of the individual should be documented in the record. Correspondence sent or received should be logged in an agency approved fashion, along with an interpretation, if appropriate. Inadequate records may appear to be of no consequence until a malpractice lawsuit is filed or until a funding source demands reimbursement for services billed but not properly documented. Then the accuracy and completeness of the record becomes a vital issue.

Accepted Progress Notes Format

Two formats for progress note documentation are commonly used in substance related disorder treatment, Subjective – Objective – Assessment – Plan (SOAP) and Data – Assessment – Plan (DAP). SOAP was developed for use in hospital settings and specifies what information is directly taken from the individuals about their condition and what is "objective" information, such as lab test results or observed symptoms. DAP combines the information gathered in both the S and O portions of SOAP into one statement(s), called Data. The following is a brief description of each, as well as an example written both ways.

SOAP Format[2]

Subjective	The individual's expression of condition, pain, complaints, reactions, etc.	S = Individual arrived complaining of headache and feelings of ear. Individual states "I'm scared."
Objective	The evidence of tests, lab finds and observations.	O = Individual has completed all paperwork for admission to treatment.
Assessment	The clinician's evaluation of the situation – professional judgment based on subjective and objective elements.	A = Individual needs reassurance about decision to enter treatment.
Plan	The course of treatment chosen.	P = Shore orientation video and discuss admission process.

Fig. 3

DAP Format[3]

Data	The individual's expression of condition, pain, complaints, reactions, etc.	D= Individual arrived complaining of headache and feelings of ear. Individual states "I'm scared." Individual has completed all paperwork for admission to treatment.
Assessment	The clinician's evaluation of the situation – professional judgment based on subjective and objective elements.	A = Individual needs reassurance about decision to enter treatment.
Plan	The course of treatment chosen.	P = Shore orientation video and discuss admission process.

Fig. 4

Both systems follow essentially the same format. What is going on with or being reported by the individual? What evidence for or against that perception is available? What can or should be done about it, based on professional knowledge? Using a format such as the ones described above serves three useful functions:

- Aids the clinician in formulating his or her thoughts
- Facilitates consistent notes throughout the record
- Provides others with a view into how the clinician came to their recommendation

What Progress Notes Should Not Include

- Opinions, value judgments and assumptions, unless clearly stated as such, as in "assessment"
- Others' names

What Progress Notes Should Include

- Date, time, and duration (length of session)
- Types of contact or service that were provided, for example: individual, group or conjoint session; consultation with physicians, therapists and other professionals
- Meetings with family, employers, or outside providers
- Peer reviews involving status changes and case conferences or staffing sessions - always state the reason for meeting and outcome
- Notes related to the Service Plan, recording progress or lack thereof
- Individual Service Plan review at staffing meeting(s) and any subsequent revisions or other outcomes from meeting
- Change in service activity, including the date of and reason for change and new activity and/or planned interventions
- Medication changes and updates
- Refusal of services/intervention(s), including the date services refused and circumstances, the staff member's immediate follow-up and the resulting interventions, contract or suspension
- Receipt, denial or substantive change in benefits from a third party payer, including the date of change and reason(s) and plans for appeal (if appropriate)
- Any change in program status
- Significant positive behaviors/progress
- Time spent away from the program (e.g., holidays and vacations)
- Discharge, including the date and reason, placement and follow-up plans
- Follow-up conducted in the case of a failure to show or an unexpected discharge
- Unusual incidents and behaviors

What Progress Notes Require

- Confidentiality – no additional individual's names
- Up-to-date and organized
- Contents in reverse chronological order (most recent page on top if paper record.)
- Notes written when services provided, and duration of services
- Clinical services and interventions
- Regular progress towards goals and objectives
- Record of all significant clinical events
- Reviews and revisions to the Individual Service Plan
- Provide justification for continued service, e.g. goals not met or interventions not carried out
- Staff signature, title and date

Documentation Oversights and Errors
(and how they are negatively interpreted in court)

- Correction fluid in a paper record – Why did they change this? Is there something being hidden?
- Out of sequence notes – Why wasn't this written when it happened? Did someone forget? What are they covering up?
- Different color ink in a single entry in a paper record – Somebody changed something here? Someone else wrote/signed this? Multiple authors?
- Missing, wrong or changed dates – Not clear when care was given. Staff didn't know what they were doing?
- Notes lacking content, vague or conflicting information, no follow-up – Was the staff competent to treat the individual?

- Lack of proper authentication – Was care given by qualified staff? Doubts about credentials of staff?
- Blank lines – Is something important missing?

Writing Tips for Progress Notes
Reality Checks

- If the clinician is out sick, on vacation or kidnapped by aliens, someone else will need to pick up where the clinician left off. Can they understand what's been happening, relying solely on the written record?
- After the clinical supervisor or an outside reviewer has examined the notes, what will the review say? Would an insurance company or Medicaid pay for the service based on the record?
- The record will be subpoenaed and read aloud in court. A lawyer will interrogate the clinician and the jury will reach a verdict based on what's been written. The clinician's own professional qualifications and competencies may be in question.
- The individual asks to see his or her record and subsequently reads the case record.
- Is this record a reflection of my abilities and of the organization?
- How would the clinician feel if this was the record of their personal care?

Conciseness Tips

- Write in plain English. Amaze readers with clarity and brevity, not literary aspirations. Don't use big words when small ones will do, don't use obscure words when everyday words suffice. A progress note is not a progress novel. "Quality not Quantity."

- "Just the facts ma'am." It's unnecessary and a waste of your valuable time to transcribe an event. Describe the essence of what occurred, not "he said," "I said," etc. If the exact words are pertinent to your report, then put them in quotes.
- Include only necessary details. Remember that when someone else reads what you've written, excessive detail can confuse the reader and distract him or her from the important points you're documenting.
- Keep sentences short.
- Avoid unneeded words. Make sure each word is necessary.
- Put action in your writing. Avoid passive verbs.
- Reexamine your writing: make sure a reader can't make something out of your writing that you didn't intend.

Do's of Case Record Documentation

- DO read the previous progress notes on your individual before meeting with them and before writing your own progress notes.
- DO have the individual's name on every page.
- DO use blue ink and write neatly and legibly so others can read what you wrote.
- DO date, time, and sign each entry.
- DO describe reported symptoms accurately. Use the individual's words when these words are helpful in describing symptoms.
- DO use accepted abbreviations wherever possible.
- DO document action taken following indication of a need for action (i.e. show resolution and follow-up).
- DO be definite. Substantiate with facts and/or descriptions.

Don'ts of Case Record Documentation

- DON'T use pencil or correction fluid ("white out").
- DON'T erase: draw a line through the entry, write "error" and initial.
- DON'T use medical terms unless you're sure of their exact meaning.
- DON'T leave blank lines. Write "N/A" or draw a line through the entry.
- DON'T write biased or vague statements such as "appears restless." Describe the behavior: e.g., "pacing," "in and out of his chair numerous times during the hour," etc.
- DON'T skip lines between entries.
- DON'T backdate, tamper with, or add notes to previously written ones. Use "late entry" or "addendum" if necessary.
- DON'T begin writing until you check to make sure you have the right case record.
- DON'T record activities in advance.
- DON'T wait until the end of your shift to record.
- DON'T rely on your memory; write notes as quickly as possible after the service is delivered.
- DON'T document for anyone else, especially for actions performed by another staff person, unless that person reviews and signs off on the entry.
- DON'T throw away progress notes that have errors on them. Mark the error.

Chapter Review

· What function do case records play in effective service

· How important is the accuracy of the record? Why?

· Name five common mistakes in record keeping.

Notes

[1]   http://www.popsci.com/technology/article/2012-09/ask-geek_how-can-i-permanently-delete-my-computer-files, accessed 17 June 2014

[2] Care Communications, The Record That Defends Itself, 4th Ed, 1989

[3] Adapted from a presentation by Miller, Karlyn-Lynn, 1996 CARF Winter Conference

CHAPTER 3

Confidentiality and Privacy

"Without trust, words become the hollow sound of a wooden gong. With trust, words become life itself."

— *John Harold*

Most clinicians understand that the foundation of any therapeutic relationship is trust. Establishing and maintaining trust in an insecure and unfamiliar environment is a challenge. Laws protecting confidentiality make the clinician's job easier and help the individual to function as a trusting person. The profession of chemical dependency counseling has its roots in Alcoholics Anonymous (AA). From its early times, AA insisted on anonymity for its members. But this was based on tradition and custom more than anything else. As chemical dependency counseling emerged as a profession, more laws and regulations were created to protect the person being served. (Note: the term patient is used throughout this chapter to conform to the language used in the regulation)

History, Regulation & HIPAA

After the epidemic drug use of the 1960s, drug and alcohol treatment was viewed as a necessity. The promise of confidentiality was thought to be an enticement to treatment: not only would the patient be protected against the stigma but he/she would also be protected from prosecution for using an illegal substance. Although laws were on the books in many states, Congress thought this issue was important enough to call for federal legislation and so the federal regulation, now known as 42 CFR, Part 2, came into being.

Since those regulations were written, another set of regulations were developed that also affect the confidentiality of case records. Chapter 45 of the Federal Regulations commonly known as Health Insurance Portability and Accountability Act (HIPPA or the Privacy Rule) applies to "covered entities" which are health plans, health care clearinghouses and health care providers who transmit health information in electronic form (i.e., via computer-based technology) in connection with transactions. HIPAA transactions that a substance abuse treatment program might engage in include: submission of claims to or coordination of benefits with health plans, inquiries to health plans regarding eligibility, coverage or benefits or status of health care claims.

Also covered by the regulations are transmission of enrollment and other information related to payment to health plans and referral certification and authorization (i.e., requests for review of health care to obtain an authorization for providing health care or requests to obtain authorization for referring an individual to another health care provider). For programs that follow the more restrictive regulations historically applied to chemical dependency programs, HIPAA is generally covered. To comply with the Privacy Rule authorization requirements, the consent must also contain a statement reflecting the ability or inability of the substance abuse treatment program to condition service on whether the patient signs the form. There are a few additional items required, such as release logs, copies of releases to the patient and retention of signed forms, which should be implemented in addition to the regulations discussed below. It is recommended that clinicians be familiar with both regulations.

Summary of Chapter 42 CFR, Part 2

Federal regulations protecting the confidentiality of alcohol and drug abuse records were initially authorized by section 408 of the Drug Abuse Prevention, Treatment, and Rehabilitation Act in 1975. Since then that section has been amended and transferred under the Public Health Service Act in 1987 and continues to be codified in Chapter 42, Code of Federal Regulations, Part 2. Those changes clarify many requirements and endeavor to simplify their administration. In general, these regulations attempt to strike a balance between protecting the confidentiality of those individuals treated for chemical dependency and the need for disclosure of patient information. Patient information may include coordination of treatment, audit, evaluation, research needs, and medical emergency situations, as well as the needs to protect others from threats or the execution of criminal justice. The regulations now apply only to programs that specialize, 1) in whole or in part, in providing alcohol or drug abuse treatment or diagnosis and referral and 2) receive any form of federal assistance, either directly or indirectly.

Restrictions

The restrictions on disclosure apply to any information, recorded or not, that identifies the patient as a chemical abuser, either directly or indirectly, including records of the identity, diagnosis, prognosis of, or services provided to the patient. Even the presence of a patient in a specialized program, directly or indirectly, cannot be disclosed. See figure 5, next page.

The General Rule

The program may not disclose any information about any individual

Exemptions

Communications not considered disclosures:
Internal communications
Business Associate Agreement
No Individual Identifiers
Conditions permitting limited disclosures:
Abuse and neglect
Crime on program premises or against program personnel
Medical emergency
Court order and subpoena
Research/audit

Proper Consent Form

Program Name
Individual Name
Purpose/need
Extent/nature
How information is to be transmitted
Individual signature
Date
Written disclosure of prohibition of redisclosure

Disclosure Permitted

To assist in diagnosis, treatment or rehabilitation
To central registry
To legal counsel
To family and others close to individual
To third-party payors and funding sources
To employers and employment agencies
To criminal justice system
In other cases where consent is freely given, no substantial harm is foreseen to the
relationship between the individual and the program and disclosure is not harmful to the individual

Prohibition on Redisclosure

Caution
This information has been disclosed to you form records whose confidentiality is protected by
Federal Law. Federal regulations (42 CFR, Part 2) prohibit you from making any further disclosure
of it without specific written consent of the person to who it pertains, or other wise permitted by
the regulations. A general authorization for the release of medical or other information is not
sufficient of this purpose.

Fig. 5

Disclosures of Patient Information

Under most circumstances disclosures may be made only if the patient first signs a consent form that is specific to the nature and purpose of such disclosures. A written consent must include:

- The name of the program or person releasing the information
- To whom the disclosure is being made
- The name of the patient
- How much and what type of information to be revealed
- The signature of the patient and, when required for a minor (or for the incompetent or deceased patient), the signature of an authorized person
- The date of the signature
- An explanation that the consent can be revoked at any time (except after the fact of disclosure)
- An expiration date (no longer than reasonably serving the purpose)

A general medical release where "any and all information" may be disclosed is not sufficient to meet the requirements of this regulation.

Think of it this way – the patient decides. The patient decides who gets the information and the patient may place limits on the amount of information to be released. The patient's consent to release information must be in writing and placed in the case file.

The general rule for clinicians and others who work in a facility governed by this regulation is "when in doubt, don't release information."

Redisclosure

The law requires that a warning against redisclosure must be attached to any information that is released. This warning is to inform the person or program receiving the information that the information may not be shared with any other persons or programs without the expressed permission of the patient. The revised law does allow the patient to generically designate more than one program/person for disclosure. Redisclosure by a receiving party may be authorized if specified; otherwise redisclosure is restricted; and in most circumstances the material disclosed should be clearly marked with an explanation of the protections of confidentiality, as stated above. The regulations also require programs to give patients a written summary of the confidentiality law.

Exceptions To Confidentiality

Whether or not the patient gives consent, disclosure of protected information is allowed under some circumstances: to medical personnel as necessary to meet a medical emergency; to those qualified to conduct research, management audits, financial audits, or program evaluation. Redisclosure is prohibited. An appropriate court order after assessing good cause (weighing public good against injury to the patient) may allow disclosures without consent under certain circumstances. In such cases, there must be appropriate limitations to provide safeguards against unrestricted disclosures. Also, confidential information cannot be used to execute criminal charges unless authorized by court order. All such restrictions remain in effect even if the individual ceases to be a patient.

Information Exchange

The regulations allow the mutual exchange of information within and between the armed forces and the health care components of the Veterans Administration. They also allow such exchange of information between program staff within the program or to an "entity" having direct administrative control over the program, such as a larger facility of which the alcohol and drug unit may be a part. There must be a need for such information for the purposes of providing treatment services (e.g. record keeping, accounting) for patients. Information should never be disclosed unless there is a need to know.

Criminal Actions

The restrictions of disclosure in these regulations do not apply to reports from program staff to law enforcement officers that are directly related to the commission or threat of a crime on the premises or against program personnel. Such reports should be limited to the circumstances of the incident, including the patient status of the individual being reported, his or her name and address and last known whereabouts. The report should also include to which individual the disclosure was made; the date and time of the disclosure; and the nature of the emergency. If the report was to the Food and Drug Administration (FDA), include error in product safety as well. As mentioned previously, other kinds of exceptions allowing for release of information without consent also exist. The regulations govern in detail when and to what extent disclosure can be made for purposes of audit, evaluation, and research. The regulations can be referred to when entering into such services and need not be enumerated here.

Court Orders

In the case of court orders, an attorney should first be consulted. Not all judicial proceedings aimed at gaining access to treatment records are sufficient to allow for release of information. Such devices as a subpoena should be resisted unless an appropriate court order is also entered. In general, such a court order cannot compel disclosure, but does authorize it. A court order accompanied by a subpoena can compel disclosure. Also, no state law may either authorize or compel any disclosure prohibited by these regulations. Such state laws may, however, add further restrictions protecting the rights of confidentiality.

Suspected Child Abuse

In addition to these exceptions, the reporting of suspected child abuse or neglect is allowed without resort to court order or written consent. Other devices for allowing disclosure without consent (such as entering a qualified service organization agreement, or reporting a medical emergency to medical personnel) are also unnecessary in the case of reporting child abuse or neglect to the appropriate state or local authorities. The federal confidentiality law does not conflict with state mandates to report such suspected abuse.

Penalties

If the regulations are violated, the law provides maximum penalties of $500 for the first offense and $5,000 for subsequent offenses. The 1987 revision of the code narrows the jurisdiction for legal action against violations of the code somewhat. Ordinarily, reports of violations should be directed to the U.S. Attorney of the appropriate judicial district in which the violation took place. In the case of a designated methadone program, legal action is executed by the Regional Office of the Food and Drug Administration (FDA). Civil action by an aggrieved person may be taken regardless of the application of the law.

Organizations Affected

It should be noted that these regulations (42CFR) do not cover programs that are not in some way federally assisted. This is true even if the individual patient is benefiting from federal support. However, federal assistance is broadly defined. An alcohol or drug abuse program is federally assisted if:

- It is in any way conducted directly or by contract, etc., by any department or agency of the United States.
- It is being carried out under authorization granted by any agency of the United States including but not limited to: certified provider under the Medicare program; authorization to conduct methadone treatment; registered to dispense controlled substances for the treatment of alcohol or drug abuse.
- It receives funds from a federal department or agency, or is conducted by state or local government that itself receives federal support.
- It is given assistance by the Internal Revenue Service for special tax consideration.

In effect, then, these regulations cover the vast majority of treatment programs specializing in the treatment of alcohol and drug abuse. Of course third party payers, administrative entities, and the like, who receive information from federally assisted programs are also governed by these regulations, whether or not they are federally assisted. Also, those persons receiving such information and notified of redisclosure restrictions are also governed by the regulations.

Disclosure of Information Relating to Minors

When the patient is a minor (less than 18 or as otherwise specified by state law), disclosure cannot be made even to a parent or guardian without the minor's consent, even for reimbursement. Of course, a program can deny treatment, unless mandated by State law. Even where State law requires both the minor's and parent or guardian's consent to treatment, disclosure of application for treatment cannot be made to the parent without the minor's consent. Any consent for disclosure of patient information will require both parent and minor's consent. A parent or guardian may be notified without consent when the minor lacks capacity for rational choice because of age or physical/mental condition and there is potential threat to life or well-being. Only the facts relevant to potentially reducing this threat may be communicated and the program director or administrator may make this judgment.

Other Exemptions

The law also provides for exemptions for those deemed to be incompetent by the courts. The person authorized under state law to act in the patient's behalf may then give consent. Where such incompetence has not been adjudicated, or the patient is not a minor, and medical condition of the patient prevents his or her action, the program director may exercise right of consent for the sole purpose of third party payment. In the case of medical emergency, necessary information may be communicated to appropriate medical personnel. In this case, upon disclosure, program personnel must document in writing to which personnel and facility and from which individual the disclosure was made; the date and time of the disclosure; and the nature of the emergency (or error in product safety, if the report was to the FDA). As mentioned previously, other kinds of exceptions allowing for release of information without consent also exist. The regulations govern in detail when and to what extent disclosure can be made for purposes of audit, evaluation, and research. The regulations can be referred to when entering into such services and need not be enumerated here.

Length of Prohibition on Disclosure

The law is regrettably (if necessarily) unwieldy and complex but it attempts to establish a reasonable balance between practical needs for flow of information and the protection of the rights of privacy of the individual. In the long run, it will prove to be helpful to programs and individual practitioners to have an in-depth knowledge of the regulations so that we save our patients from unnecessary invasions of privacy. Our knowledge may help us to avoid litigation but above all, we protect our patients' privacy, not because of potential sanctions but because it is the right thing to do.

One important caveat: don't ever forget that the clinician is bound to honor confidentiality in perpetuity, and that means forever!

Chapter Review

- Who is covered by the Federal Regulations regarding confidentiality?

- What is the "general rule" regarding confidentiality?

- What are the exceptions to the "general rule?"

- How long must a person adhere to the confidentiality regulations?

CHAPTER 4

Substance Related Disorder Psychosocial Assessment

"There is nothing about a caterpillar which would suggest that it will turn into a butterfly."

— *R. Buckminster Fuller*

Performing an accurate assessment is the essential first step in the treatment of the individual. It is also the foundation from which the remainder of the treatment services is built. A person who arrives for an assessment may be appearing for the first time in the social or chemical dependency service system. A moderate level of anxiety, defensiveness and even hostility is common. If you plan for these reactions you can put the person at ease.

Setting the Stage for Success

It is important to remember that an individual who walks into a treatment setting is there for a reason. Something or someone in their life has raised the question of their relationship with alcohol and drugs. This does <u>not</u> mean that they have a problem with substances beyond that particular event or relationship. Be careful to look at all the factors related to their substance use.

Often the assessment appointment is the first face to face contact. A screening telephone call may have been conducted to gather basic information prior to the appointment. An important cue to the handling of your interview is the reason and source of the referral. A person who comes in as a result of a court order may need a different approach than a person who claims to be self-referred. It is best to treat all individuals as though they are showing very good judgment in coming in to seek assistance. After all, even in the case of a legal referral a person likely has other choices – perhaps not desirable ones for most, but choices.

Building Rapport

Building rapport with an individual is essential to good information gathering and beginning the therapeutic process. There is a special skill in being able to assist people to ventilate their feelings, if necessary, and to encourage the voicing of concerns regarding the outcome of the assessment. Often, answering this uneasiness at the outset can create a more comfortable session. Asking open-ended questions regarding the person's expectations is helpful. Beware of a totally open ended style for your information gathering; until you have acquired good skills in discerning what information has most importance it may be difficult to sort personal data on the fly. Carefully explaining the assessment process, your understanding of their possible embarrassment or reluctance to answer some questions and the need for candor can help to ease some of the individual's anxiety.

Assessing Literacy

An important factor in weighing the information that you receive from individuals is their level of literacy. Some questions to ask yourself or other staff are: Were they able to fill out the forms themselves? Do the answers reflect understanding of the questions? Is the handwriting legible? Did they need help in the form's completion? What was the degree of that help – mere assistance in understanding, or actual completion by someone else? Investigate this area with care, as it can be an area of shame for some individuals. Embarrassment and shame are barriers to a productive interview. Be aware of the person who says "I forgot my glasses." He or she may be unable to read or read at the level of your forms. On an agency level, it is important that the intake forms you use have been tested by a sample of your population being served and that people have had the opportunity to give feedback on the ease of use of those forms.

Resistance

The reason for this assessment plays a big role in the development of the individual's resistance. Even the most willing participants may balk at giving you certain information. Most individuals become resistant at some point or another in the interview. Anticipate this and prepare to "roll" with the resistance. If an individual is reluctant to disclose information, simply note that and move on. If your recommendation meets with resistance, do not attempt to convince or push the individual into a particular opinion or option. Pick your battles and make sure that your facts and attitudes, as well as their symptoms, are accurate and relevant. Motivational interviewing techniques developed by William Miller, et al, are essential in setting the proper tone to encourage the individual to seek appropriate additional help when needed.

Boundary Setting

Set appropriate boundaries with your individual. This refers to both rapport and resistance. Maintain a stance of helping in a cooperative way. Encourage the person to take care of arrangements and responsibilities for themselves when possible. While much treatment can involve what is termed "benevolent coercion," attempting to force an individual into compliance of any type is unethical and is likely to backfire. State the consequences of non-compliance clearly. Writing them down is often most effective, providing that the person fully understands prior to your written confirmation. Always discuss your recommendations with the individual when possible.

Appropriate boundaries may also need to be set with the referent. In some cases, depending upon the circumstances, a clinician might be asked to give out information without a proper release of information form. A clinician may also be asked to render an assessment decision that is not supported by the data that has been gathered. Be clear about your professional responsibilities to the individual. An incorrect diagnosis can carry considerable penalties and/or consequences for the individual concerned and also affects your credibility. Your reputation is one of your most important assets and should be carefully safeguarded. Ethical violations may also have legal consequences; be sure you are clear and accurate in your reporting.

Gathering Information
Rapport, Again

If the individual has filled out some of the intake information themselves, always go over that information with them to check its completeness and accuracy. Reading abilities, as well as anxiety about the interview, can affect validity. Going over the information the person provided is also an easy way to establish rapport. For example, you can say: "I see here you have two children, 9 and 11. Are they soccer fans like my kids?" Look for commonalities between you and the individual, such as, "I used to live over near Lake Street and went to the coffee shop every morning on the way to work. Is that coffee shop still there?" Be vague about personal matters and keep to light topics of conversation at this stage. This can assist the person in becoming more comfortable with sharing information with you. The rule of thumb is to gather the least sensitive information first and save the most difficult probing for later when the individual has acquired some level of comfort with you and the surroundings.

Take a Holistic Approach

After gathering demographic information, including history, it is important to bear in mind the primary focus of the assessment – determining whether or not the person is chemically dependent. Remember that particularly in the early stages, a substance related disorder is generally manifested through life problems and the consequences of drug or alcohol use rather than chronic signs and symptoms. As current and historical information is gathered, be sensitive to these common themes: chronic health problems, especially of the types listed on the intake and assessment form and frequent legal, family or vocational problems. An assessment of the current risk of withdrawal and the risk of additional physical problems is also important. Untreated physical problems can increase relapse potential. Various instruments used to clarify withdrawal risk, such as the Clinical Institute Withdrawal Assessment for Alcohol, Revised (CIWA-Ar), can be very informative and help to give the individual unbiased feedback about their condition. Copies are downloadable from various internet sources.

Repetition

The use of repetition can be helpful. This applies particularly to questions that may be of special importance, such as assessing physical status. Ask the same question several times in different ways. "When was the last time you saw a doctor?" "The date of your last physical was when?" "When you last saw the doctor in (name month), he said what again about your stomach?" Use the "Columbo" approach. Remember him? Colombo was the 1970s TV detective played by Peter Falk who always seemed to forget or fumble, but all the time knew exactly what he was doing. He did this by feigning puzzlement and in the process, he showed them the inconsistency of their actions. His only tools were modesty, logic and observation. He dealt with sophisticated people who believed they can get away with murder. In the end, admissions are graceful; there are no fights, no raising of voices — it's more like checkmate. No one argues with the conclusion. You'll be surprised how many times you will get different answers or uncover important information. Remember, substance related disorder is a brain disorder. Addicted individuals are deluded about how drugs and alcohol have affected their lives, and repetition and direct feedback can help them begin to see the magnitude of these changes.

Paraphrasing

Repeat back to the individual what you thought you heard. Develop a habit of repeating, especially important information. It may be tempting to hurry to complete the information gathering, but poor decisions can be based on what someone thought they heard. Paraphrasing also helps in the feedback process for the individual by emphasizing areas that are of particular concern. (see Emphasis, below)

Emphasis

Providing emphasis on key points when giving feedback can be a tool to help the individual self-diagnose. Repetition of essential diagnostic criteria, e.g., loss of control, can help disable the "built-in forgetter." Try a summarizing feedback comment like "Let me see if I've got this right: you went to visit your in-laws and told your wife that you would not drink. Three hours later you had consumed eight beers and argued with your father in law. Is that correct?" Don't ask for an explanation or you'll get one, generally well steeped in denial. Just leave it and move on. Use this repetition sparingly in the initial phases of the session, or the individual may notice your emphasis and not disclose as completely.

Collateral Sources

Whenever possible, obtain information from other sources – spouses, school records, police reports and employers' performance records. Use judgment when weighing this information as to its validity. In the case of police reports, watch closely for a high Breathalyzer reading coupled with "good" performance on physical tests – a sure sign of tolerance. Conversely, a low Blood Alcohol Level with poor physicals could mean other drugs are involved. In reading the police report and discussing the incident with the individual, look for dissimilarities. Sometimes an individual will eventually disclose to you that they have no recollection of the incident at all.

When using others' verbal reports, rather than documents, listen closely for specific data. A person's feelings, while important, are less effective for your purposes than verifiable data, for example the individual was late four times this month with no excuse. One standard to use is: does my individual's perception of reality match or at least seem similar to that of a recognized authority or a close relative or friend?

Weighing Information
Testing Validity

Always use diagnostic testing in which you have confidence, but remember that it is only a paper and pencil (or computer generated) test and no substitute for clinical judgment. A toxic individual may answer a test in a very erratic way. Some tests work better than others. No diagnostic test is perfect. Most tests are not normed with an average standard on all populations nor do they take into account low literacy levels. Use healthy skepticism when assessing test results. Be sure that your skills in giving the test are up to the necessary levels. Never use a test in lieu of an interview or your own clinical skills.

Use of Short and Long-term Information

The individual may deny any recent problems despite a long history of difficulties. What has happened to change things? Have things really changed? Have the individual's life circumstances changed in a way that minimizes any overt problems with alcohol or drugs? If the individual's difficulties are recent in origin, what is different now? Generally in addiction there is a discernible pattern that progresses over time and the individual's life events will reflect a pattern of deterioration.

Collateral Information

Collateral information is what is obtained from sources other than the individual you are assessing. These could include parents, spouse, employer, the justice system, police reports or other information. The information may be verbal or written and should be included in your assessment decision, along with any comments you may have regarding its validity. What do these sources have to gain or lose by giving you information? A spouse may have concerns regarding loss of employment or retaliation by his or her spouse. A defense attorney may wish to portray the individual in the best light possible. What was the source's purpose for gathering or reporting the information in the first place? It may have been to convict on a Driving Under the Influence (DUI) charge for example, or to make an Employee Assistance Program (EAP) referral. Consider the information from collateral sources in light of the source's motivation.

Assessment of Information
Clarity of Terms

Many practitioners use some terms interchangeably: "assessment" and "evaluation" are two examples. Often we forget that individuals, even those who have a long history of treatment, do not know our clinical terms. Be certain that the recommendations you are making are clear to the individual. Avoid jargon, such as "clean" and "sober." These are common terms to clinicians and recovering people but may be misinterpreted by others. When discussing drug and alcohol use with an individual, make sure you are clear what you mean: all use, no matter what type, and a definite time frame.

Usefulness of Information

Take nothing for granted. Ask questions. Depending on the person, much time can be wasted getting information that has little or no bearing on the diagnostic statement. Have a goal in mind when you ask a question. Depending on the communication style of the individual, open-ended questions may generate too much information, or not enough. Crisis generated information and behavior may be suspect. How a person responds during a crisis, such as getting a DUI, may not tell you much about how they might respond to day to day activities. Extraordinary events may produce uncharacteristic behavior.

In the assessment the goal is to gather information to support recommendations for or against treatment, with initial recommendations for modalities and lengths of stay, as needed. Themes are likely to emerge and implications for further planning may be evident. These should be addressed in the assessment or assessment summary. The treating practitioner, not the assessment professional, should design the full Individual Service Plan in collaboration with the person being treated.

Signs and Symptoms

Diagnosis is made using the identified signs and symptoms reported by the individual. Signs are better than symptoms. A sign is something observable or verifiable by another. Your observation can be biased, but generally is more accurate than your report of a symptom. Although an individual complains of "anxiety" you notice fresh needle tracks on his arms. Symptoms are states that the individual reports; a complaint of "depression" for example, is a symptom. Symptoms can be distorted by both the individual's perception and yours.

Assessment Summary

There are several reasons to write an assessment summary interpreting the information you have gathered as well as your impression of and recommendations for the individual. The most obvious and practical one is to allow other practitioners to easily access the information regarding the individual: either verbally, as in a clinical staffing, or as an introduction prior to treatment admission. Assessment summaries can be done in a variety of formats, but should include the essential information about the individual, e.g., general description, diagnosis with rationale for it and recommendations for treatment. The individual's perception of the problem and their strengths and needs are also important.

Too often, assessment summaries are simply a recounting of the information gathered. A good summary utilizes the knowledge and skill of the practitioner to synthesize the information into an understandable account and a clear recommendation for the individual. It is important to remember that if the individual and their family could have solved this crisis without your aid, they would have. Being clear about why you are recommending a certain course is as important as what is being recommended.

Neal Adams, M.D. and Diane Grieder, M.Ed. state in their excellent book *Treatment Planning for Person-Centered Care, Shared Decision Making for Whole Health*: "The ability of the provider to integrate data into understanding, and the sharing of this insight and perspective with the individual and family, is often in and of itself a powerful intervention. It is the essence of empathy, a key ingredient of successful helping relationships. The provider is not merely a sponge absorbing facts and detail but rather a skilled partner working in collaboration with the individual and family.

Sharing the understanding and formulation that emerges provides an opportunity to further that alliance."[1]

Assessment Summary

The following is an example of an assessment summary which incorporates use of placement criteria dimensions.

Alice M. Green is a 33 year-old African American female, who has been divorced twice and has no children. Ms. Green completed 10 years of education and has obtained her GED certificate. Ms. Green reports that she has "quit drinking many times" but begins again after a period of time. She is interested in eliminating the problems that are currently taking her time and resources. She would like to stabilize her job situation.

Ms. Green sought treatment at this time due to the effects and consequences of her perceived dependence on alcohol, specifically a DUI, and possible dependence on Valium. The signs and symptoms of alcohol dependence are: increased tolerance, failed attempts to cut down or quit, family complaints, work problems, legal problems, and continued use despite adverse consequences.

The assessment indicates the following:

Alcohol withdrawal risk: high due to continued use, reported symptoms of withdrawal and current use of Valium. Potential exists for benzodiazepine withdrawal and she should be carefully monitored for delayed withdrawal symptoms.

Biomedical conditions or complications: chronic stomach complaints that should be investigated by a physician. High blood pressure has been diagnosed and Ms. Green is currently taking medication for same.

Emotional, behavioral or cognitive conditions: reported anxiety and panic attacks, currently treated with Valium by her primary care physician. Cessation of Valium may temporarily increase frequency of these attacks. The psychological history includes no previous treatment for either psychological or addiction problems. Ms. Green reports some memory loss but appears to have adequate impulse control when not drinking. Her present spiritual orientation is likely to support recovery because she states that she "believes in God."

Readiness to Change: treatment acceptance is fair at this time due to legal difficulties and her desire to resolve them. Ms. Green's current motivation for this treatment is primarily due to pending DUI, and she appears to be a good candidate for deferred prosecution.

Continued Use or Continued Problem Potential: Based on previous use history and the current assessment, potential for continued use is high at this time. She expresses a serious concern regarding her ability to function, and to work, without use of Valium, at minimum.

Recovery/Living Environment: does not support recovery in several aspects. Her current living situation, with her boyfriend of six months, may include domestic violence. Her boyfriend drinks regularly and Ms. Green has complained about his actions when drinking. She works at a bar as a singer and her entire social network consists of people who drink. Her employer has complained about her drinking. She has failed to maintain a steady "gig" since 2006. The social assessment indicates a family history of substance related disorder /abuse. Ms. Green's father is described by her as an "active alcoholic."

Findings and Recommendation:

Our findings, including diagnostic testing, support a diagnosis of substance use disorder alcohol use disorder – severe. Anxiolytic use disorder should be ruled out. The following treatment modalities and lengths of stay are recommended until Ms. Green has made satisfactory progress and is thus likely to be able to continue recovery at a less intensive level of care: Intoxication management (medically managed) 3 -7 days dependent upon medical screening and Valium reduction schedule. Attend and complete intensive residential treatment for 14-21 days, followed by recovery house for 3-9 months.

Ms. Green should make progress in these skills, behaviors or social conditions prior to transfer to a less intensive level of care: 1. Achieve withdrawal management stabilization, 2. Acknowledge need for long-term recovery program, 3. Develop long-term recovery plan.

(Signed)
Chemical Dependency Professional
Date

Making Individual Recommendations

When a recommendation is made to enter a treatment program, always explain the structure of the program, the course of treatment you are recommending, why you feel that it is important, and what you hope the individual will gain from completing this course of treatment. If you have materials such as brochures or information sheets on your program or other facilities, provide those for the individual to take away. Writing down your recommendations, including self-help, doctor's visits, etc., are important, but don't give the individual too much to handle in a short time. Give the individual as many choices as possible within your recommendation, but also attempt to get a commitment to follow through on at least a portion of your recommendation by a set date. If appropriate, set a check back appointment or phone call as soon as practical.

When writing a recommendation for a legal entity, provide as little information as possible to support your recommendation and meet their requirements. Your correspondence with the court becomes public record. You must have a release of information to communicate the information, but that doesn't mean you should provide each detail of the individual's life. Err on the side of non-disclosure. You can always respond to questions, should they be asked. You can use your summary, if appropriate, as a beginning and pare down the information. Remember that your relationship with the individual is based on trust. Be sure that they understand what will be disclosed, and to whom.

Chapter Review

- Why are building rapport and good communication skills essential to a good assessment?

- What are some ways to check on the validity of the information that you gather?

- What are some of the uses of an assessment summary?

Notes

[1] Neal Adams, M.D. and Diane Grieder, M.Ed., Treatment Planning for Person-Centered Care, Shared Decision Making for Whole Health, Copyright 2014

CHAPTER 5

Patient Placement Criteria

"All we see of someone at any moment is a snapshot of their life, there in riches or poverty, in joy or despair. Snapshots don't show the million decisions that led to that moment."

— *Richard Bach*

Criteria Development

Clinicians make dozens of decisions during the course of a day. Many of our decisions affect other people's lives in important ways. Some of our decisions need to be based on the collective pre-existing judgments found in such sources as laws, regulations, administrative codes, diagnostic manuals and agency policies and procedures. For instance, we often ask ourselves:

- "What does confidentiality suggest about the fact that I need information about my individual?"
- "What does our agency policy say about the fact that my individual attended only half the required support groups this week?"

• "What signs and symptoms are required to meet the eligibility requirements for a particular insurance company?"

Sometimes we have memorized the criteria and sometimes we look them up. Assuming the criteria have been well thought out and tested, their use can guide us in our decision making, giving us some assurance that we are making judgments that are consistent with professional standards.

One of the most commonly used set of criteria in substance related disorder treatment is the American Society of Addiction Medicine (ASAM) Criteria. A number years ago, in response to feedback from insurance companies, a number of professionals nationwide collaborated to test a number of different criteria to assist with placement in substance abuse treatment. Out of these efforts a variety of different criteria were born.

ASAM Criteria provide the clinician with a unified set of guidelines to use in matching patient treatment needs with treatment services and creates a common language for use among organizations that use the same criteria. ASAM Criteria were then developed to answer the need for better communication about benefits eligibility between treatment providers and the insurance industry. Although some states have developed their own Patient Placement Criteria (PPC), the most common criteria found are those of the American Society of Addiction Medicine (ASAM). This chapter is a general overview of placement criteria and a discussion of its implications for case management.

Detailed descriptions of the levels of service, dimensions and criteria can be found in the ASAM Criteria itself.[1] This chapter is intended to encourage use of placement criteria in general rather than as a summary of the contents of the ASAM Criteria. If the reader elects to use this particular criteria, one is strongly encouraged to refer to a copy of the ASAM Criteria for more detail and clinical use.

Underlying Assumptions

Understanding the placement criteria requires an awareness of the following assumptions:

- The objectivity that the clinician uses in the assessment of substance-related disorders should be no different than other medical conditions - a mixture of objective criteria and subjective professional judgment.
- Professional judgment must be used on a case-by-case basis. ASAM Criteria, for example, contains the caveat that they are not intended, and should not be used, as a standard for the treatment of any individual. The treatment of individuals requires professional evaluation and the exercise of independent judgment on a case-by-case basis. The criteria are a format for professional decisions and a way to objectively use the same decision as others.
- The use of criteria is an evolutionary process. How they apply to the wide variety of substance related disorder services available, as well as to other health care providers, the insurance industry and the criminal justice system is an on-going scenario that will take years to fully develop. The criteria are not a set of rules carved in stone.
- The goal of the criteria is placing the individual in the most appropriate level of service based on individual needs and response to treatment goals. The treatment system is an open continuum, with an individual being able to enter at any level and move to any other level. Levels may be skipped or utilized in consecutive order. Unlike earlier versions of the ASAM Criteria, for example, treatment

services are "unbundled," i.e., the type and intensity of service are determined by the Individual Service Plan and not by limitations imposed by the treatment setting. For instance, an individual with a number of treatment needs may receive services at various levels that are appropriate for individual treatment goals. Services are not necessarily provided at the level that is most intensive.

· Based on individual needs, he or she may receive services within one agency or through referral to other providers. For example, an individual who is able to actively participate in an outpatient program, but who needs some medical assistance with depression, might be referred to another provider for that specific need. The substance disorder services continue at the first agency.

· Lack of progress in treatment at a given service level should not automatically be used as an admission criterion to another level. Individual treatment placement decisions should be made based upon a thorough assessment. The lack of progress of an individual at a particular level of service should not be attributed to the individual alone. Often there are other contributing factors, such as the appropriateness of the treatment level, quality of treatment and treatment planning, logistics and financial considerations.

· Individual needs and the goals of the Individual Service Plan should determine the ideal level of service, not program content, finances or the criminal justice system.

· In order to use the criteria, the care provider must first make an assessment that the individual meets the diagnostic criteria of a substance-related disorder using standardized and widely accepted criteria, usually the Diagnostic and Statistical Manual of Mental Disorders, Fifth Edition (DSM-5).[2]

· Criteria may encourage the use of self-help recovery groups, such as Alcoholics Anonymous, but such groups are not considered a formal treatment level due to the lack of "formal programming."

· ASAM Criteria, for example, recognizes that availability of appropriate services, progress in treatment and state laws may require exceptions, including the use of different criteria.

Criteria Dimensions

Dimensions are an attempt to organize the assessment of an individual's condition into a set of standardized categories that can be objectively measured. One of the terms that has been used is the biopsychosocial model, which takes a systems approach to assessment.

ASAM Criteria dimensions are lenses with which to view the individual, not convenient labels. Dimensions are an attempt to define individual needs holistically using language that can help us measure the results of our treatment. The following figure illustrates some of the different models.

Dimension 1

Acute Intoxication and/or Withdrawal refers to the withdrawal risk of the person. Although we have traditionally thought of detox as being done in a residential setting, medical advances now provide for detox at any level. For example, an individual who is at mild risk for withdrawal and who has access to the office of a substance disorder physician, might satisfactorily complete the needs of this dimension without being admitted to a hospital. On the other hand, the criteria recommend a residential setting for someone with a history of severe withdrawal symptoms.

Questions to ask in Dimension 1

- "What is the individual's previous withdrawal history? This includes where and when the services were received.
- "When was the last use of mood altering substances?"
- "What substances have been used recently?"
- "Does the individual exhibit any withdrawal symptoms?"

Dimension 2

Biomedical concerns itself with the person's physical condition, particularly those conditions that may complicate substance disorder treatment. Common coexisting conditions with substance disorders are alcoholic hepatitis and cirrhosis, pancreatitis and cardiac and pulmonary diseases.

Questions to ask in Dimension 2

- "Where and when was your last physical exam?"
- "What is the name of your doctor?"
- "Are there any physical conditions (other than withdrawal) that need to be addressed or which complicate treatment?"
- "Are there chronic conditions that affect treatment?"

Dimension 3

Emotional/Behavioral conditions are those psychiatric illnesses or psychological, behavioral or emotional problems that need to be addressed or which complicate substance disorder treatment. Examples found in this Dimension are cognitive dysfunction, personality disorders, anti-social behavior and depression not induced by alcohol.

Questions to ask in Dimension 3

- "Are there current psychiatric illnesses or psychological, behavioral or emotional problems that need to be addressed or which complicate substance disorder treatment?"
- "Are there chronic conditions that affect treatment?"
- "Do any of these problems appear to be an expected part of addiction illness? Example: depression. Are any of these problems severe enough to warrant specific mental health treatment?"

Dimension 4

Treatment Acceptance/Resistance is a measure of the individual's willingness to accept and participate in treatment, the individual's willingness to change and the individual's perceived addiction problem.

Questions to ask in Dimension 4

- "What ability does the individual have to connect their substance use with the consequences?
- "What is the individual's motivation for treatment?" "For recovery in general?"
- "What is the individual's attitude toward self-help groups?"
- "What previous experiences or preconceptions does the individual have?""
- "How does the individual verbalize the concept of addiction?"
- "What level of service does the individual express a willingness to attend?" • "How does the individual express an understanding of relapse behaviors?"
- "What behaviors indicate the need for structure in treatment?"

- "What issues may impact success/entry in treatment (age, language, literacy or ethnicity)?"

Dimension 5

Relapse/Continued Use Potential is the ability of the person to recognize or understand the skills needed to prevent relapse and a measure of the risk of relapse.

Questions to ask in Dimension 5

- "What is the individual's relapse history?" Include agency, level, treatment problems and progress, and lengths of service and dates.
- "What kinds of relapse prevention training have been provided in the past?"
- "What is the impulse control ability of the individual?"
- "What preoccupation of craving symptoms does the individual have?"
- "What ability does the individual have to refuse chemicals?"
- "What are the consequences of relapse?"
- "What specific relapse prevention skills training are needed to prevent relapse in the future?"

Dimension 6

Recovery Environment refers to family members, significant others, living situations or school/work settings that support or pose a threat to treatment and/or recovery.

Questions to ask in Dimension 6

- "What are the social activities and relationships that support alcohol and other drug use?"

- "What are the social activities and relationships that support recovery?"
- "How does the individual verbalize their social support?"
- "What environmental issues are likely to impact recovery (e.g., employment, abuse, living situation, etc.)?"

Implicit in the organization of the Dimensions is the acknowledgment of spirituality in the assessment, treatment and continuity of care for substance-related disorders. The ASAM Criteria states that spirituality may even transcend each level of care. Spirituality is not explicitly a part of the dimensions due to the difficulty of providing definitions in acceptable objective, behavioral and measurable terms.

Levels of Service

ASAM Criteria contain levels of service that range from early intervention to outpatient to managed inpatient care. The key to understanding the levels is to remember that they are defined by the services provided, not necessary the physical setting or program location. In all cases we are talking about an organized and structured program with professional staff, which includes addiction treatment professionals and, when appropriate, addiction physicians. Detox services may occur in any level except Level 0.5. Attaching a level to any particular program's services should be undertaken with care.

- Early Intervention (Level 0.5) is an organized, educational service. Examples include Alcohol and Other Drug Information School programs and individual counseling that might occur in Employee and Student Assistance Programs.

- Outpatient (Level I) is a non-residential program, usually less than nine hours of service per week.
- Intensive Outpatient/Day Treatment or Partial Hospitalization (Level II) is a non-residential program.
- Residential/Inpatient (Level III) services provide a planned program in a 24-hour live-in setting for those individuals whose treatment needs require an environment with more structured interventions. The focus is in the Dimensions concerning treatment acceptance/resistance, relapse and recovery environment.

When the Criteria Are Used

Criteria are used continuously to measure the attainment of treatment goals. At admission, each dimension is assessed and the admission criteria are used to make an initial recommendation based on the services needed to meet the needs of the person's Individual Service Plan. This recommendation, while global in nature, may include placing the individual in more than one service level. The key questions at admission are: "What services are required to meet the needs of the individual person?" and "Where will these services to be provided?" While the process may seem complex at first, this strengths-based approach facilitates placement of the individual in just the right treatment setting to meet individual goals. The clinician can recommend, for example, specific treatment services that are targeted to particular goals instead of placing the individual in a generalized program that may waste time and resources.

Criteria are also used during Individual Service Plan reviews to measure attainment of treatment goals. This is one reason why Individual Service Plans must be written with measurable goals and objectives. Frequency of Individual Service Plan reviews will depend on the intensity of services provided and individual progress in attaining treatment goals. Several key questions to ask during Individual Service Plan review are: "Is the Individual Service Plan producing expected results?" and "Do the results in the Individual Service Plan indicate a change in intensity of service at this level or a change in service level?" and "If the results are less than expected, how can the Individual Service Plan be revised?" One important shift in treatment is for the clinician to look at both the individual and at the service provider when satisfactory progress toward meeting treatment goals is not achieved.

The continuous assessment of treatment goals continues until the individual meets the Discharge criteria (or, logically, the individual no longer meets the criteria for continued stay). The key question at discharge is "Has there been sufficient achievement of treatment goals or sufficient worsening of Dimensional conditions to warrant transfer to another level of service?" Note that this may include those individuals who need a more appropriate level of service due to lack of response to treatment despite staff interventions.

Using a Criteria Environment

One primary impact of criteria for the clinician is in Individual Service Planning. The assessment must be thorough and detailed to assess individual needs and goals for treatment. The assessment, though focused on substance abuse, must be multidimensional and result in a summary that addresses each criteria dimension.

Individual Service Plans must be written in behavioral terms so that goals and plans based on strengths, needs, abilities and preferences are measurable. The individual's strengths, needs and goals must flow logically from information contained in the assessment, not from pre-conceived generalizations about what individuals with substance related disorder need. Interventions that are provided by program staff to achieve individual treatment goals are based on the continuous measurement of their achievement, not "one size fits all" program content.

The chief challenges to Individual Service Planning under criteria seem to be twofold. The first is the switch to a specific focus on individual strengths, needs, abilities preferences (rather than "programs and content"). The clinician needs to ask "What specific services does my individual need to meet treatment goals?" and then "Where should these services be provided?" The second challenge is clinical writing that is behavioral-focused and measurable, as well as clear and understandable. This becomes a matter of practice and patience, and can be solved over time by the use of the suggestions that follow.

- Individual Service Plan review and team staffing of individuals on a frequent basis are essential for the value of learning, mutual support and to provide the creativity needed to use the criteria. The staff involved should help decide the frequency and format of these meetings and the decisions made should be documented.
- Each treatment team should develop a shared master book of clinical writing that works for that agency. Sentences and phrases (and whole Individual Service Plans) that are developed by the staff should be readily available for use so they can be adapted to the individual. It is much quicker to adapt a pre-written sentence than to sit at a desk trying to put the whole thing together. This is not the same thing as having pre-printed Individual Service Plans, which should be avoided.
- Providers must have clinical supervision that focuses on meaningful and consistent review of Individual Service Planning and placement decisions. This includes continual training and when appropriate corrective action.

- Forms should be as easy to use as possible. Computer software can help, especially to help reduce or eliminate duplication and to process routine letters, but is not a substitute for professional judgment.
- Conduct a thorough analysis of the entire treatment system, with line staff participation. To provide the time for treatment planning and continuous assessment, each portion of the system must be looked at to eliminate duplication and unnecessary forms.
- Finally, the use of criteria requires time, training, practice and patience. Criteria for patient treatment, like other sets of criteria we use, are tools to increase our professional judgment as well as the efficiency and effectiveness of treatment.

Chapter Review

- What are some of the reasons for the existence of ASAM Criteria? Define the dimensions.

- Define the levels.

- What is the difference between the use of the ASAM Criteria and the DSM-5?

- How does the use of criteria support more effective treatment?

Notes

[1] Mee-Lee D, Shulman GD, Fishman MJ, Gastfriend DR and Miller MM, eds. The ASAM Criteria: Treatment Criteria for Addictive, Substance-Related, and Co-Occurring Conditions, 3rd ed. Carson City, NV: The Change Companies®; 2013.

[2] American Psychiatric Association: Desk Reference to the Diagnostic Criteria from DSM-5, Arlington, VA, American Psychiatric Association, 2013

CHAPTER 6

Individualized Service Planning

"When you come to a fork in the road, take it."

— *Yogi Berra*

Person centered individual planning is a process by which clinician and individual work together to:

• Identify and rank the problems needing resolution.
• Establish agreed upon immediate and long-term goals
• Decide on a treatment process and resources needed.

Historical Origins

The Individual Service Plan or ISP, sometimes called the "care plan" or "treatment plan," has its origins in the field of medicine. It is an integral part of the entire health-care service delivery system, which includes physical health, mental health and substance related disorders.

Most of the early Individual Service Plans in the chemical dependency field were basic, look-alike plans that would fit almost every individual. This process would begin in detox, where a medical plan or protocol would be implemented. Standing orders, or treatment that is given to each patient, regardless of their individual differences, were common in many sections of medicine. These protocols commonly included medications, including over the counter ones, such as pain killers, as well as prescription medicines to ameliorate the symptoms of withdrawal. Routine vital sign monitoring was included.

When the individual was transitioned to the next level of care, generally intensive treatment of one type or another, plans of the "cookie cutter" type were often continued. As a result, individuals were uncertain as to what they were trying to accomplish while in treatment, other than to "stay sober" or "get better." Even the clinician had only vague goals and sometimes non-existent objectives. While it is true that many addicted individuals have similar sets of problems and sometimes the same goals, the look-a-like or "cookie-cutter" approach doesn't work long term as it seldom addresses individual needs. Treatment completion under this system was based on how much time elapsed between admission and discharge. Discharge criteria became a certain number of days for residential treatment and a number of hours or sessions for outpatient. In both cases time in treatment was used rather than response to individual treatment goals

Current Practice

Today, Individual Service Plans must be more precise. Plans should be specific regarding goals and interventions and must demonstrate that the individual's needs and preferences are being considered. Goals must be measurable and show clear markers that can be used to record progress. Unlike the past, today's clinicians are obliged to produce effective, high quality plans in a short period of time. Establishment of the medical necessity of treatment can be directly tied to the Individual Service Plan, and in some sophisticated systems, reimbursement is based on establishment and monitoring of the plan.

The individual's participation in this planning process is vital. Before you begin, it is important to find out what the person wants from treatment. The clinician and the individual work together and decide on the best methods to get where they want to go. In some cases, collaboration with the family on this goal setting is desirable.

The Process

If treatment is the journey, then treatment planning is the map that guides us. From time to time we adjust as changes occur and as we arrive at a single destination we look ahead to the next one. When we study our map we can see how far we've come and get a good look at how far we have to go. And so it is with the Individual Service Plan. It is a measure of progress. It shows us the way to our goals and lets us know when we have arrived. Most importantly, it reflects the needs and preferences of the individual and is tailored to their strengths and abilities.

Begin the Journey

Before we start our travels we must first decide where we'd like to go. The foundation of the Individual Service Plan is the assessment. Prioritizing the issues that have been identified during the assessment and intake process helps to decide where to go first. During this process, the individual may talk about a wide variety of issues. The clinician's job is to play detective. Which of these issues is most important? Which ones can be dealt with while this individual is in treatment? Most of the time a primary goal will become evident and this goal goes to the top of the list. Some secondary goals will show up and they can be listed only if they can be treated appropriately in your facility. Certain goals are set aside and dealt with at a later date.

A truly effective plan can deal with only a few goals. Overloading the ISP is not realistic nor is it conducive to reaching the stated goals. It is too easy to get lost. A simple plan retains its focus and both the person being served and the clinician will find it easier to follow.

Remember, the plan is not carved in stone. Just as you can adjust the direction of your journey when using a road map, you can adjust the ISP to fit the developing needs of the individual. At any time, if the plan proves to be insufficient, it can be revised or rewritten. It is essential to engage the person in the planning process and keep them engaged as revisions are made. Service planning does not occur in a vacuum. It is a joint effort between you and the person being served. Input from other staff or the treatment team is also a vital part of the process.

Developing a List

As you review the assessment to develop a goal or needs list, it is important to keep in mind which goals you are capable of accomplishing. If your long-range goal for the individual is recovery from substance related disorder then you will want to focus on issues that are current barriers to recovery. These issues, if unresolved or not addressed, may prevent the individual from achieving and maintaining sobriety. This is the beginning of a decision making process in which you separate the more emergent goals from the less time sensitive and choose the ones you will work on. The other issues may be postponed or given over to another person or agency. A good rule to follow: any goal identified in the assessment must be accounted for on the goal list. If you review all the goals and weigh their importance or urgency your priorities will become fairly obvious. Keep in mind that you or your facility may not be capable of treating some goals even though they are important or urgent. This is where deferral and referral come in.

Knowing the what, who, and when of referral is an important addition to treatment.

Obtaining information directly from another facility regarding a prior treatment episode can be time consuming and sometimes non-productive. It cannot be stressed enough, however, the value of this information in assisting the individual to identify issues leading to relapse and treatment noncompliance. If it is not possible to get written documents, a telephone call to the previous counselor may be helpful. This information should be integrated into treatment planning. Remember that information from the facility staff member will not be forthcoming without a signed release in their possession.

Setting Priorities

A tool that can be helpful in your initial prioritization is the Hierarchy of Needs, developed by Abraham Maslow[1]. Maslow posited that human beings must have their needs met in a certain order to enable them to work on needs at the next level. Maslow's Hierarchy (see figure 6) shows that first biological and physiological needs - air, food, water, shelter, warmth, sex, sleep – must be met before the individual can address needs such as protection issues: security, order, law, limits, stability. When basic needs have been met then the individual begins to notice belongingness and love needs such as being part of a group or family, having affection and relationships. Esteem needs appear to be met next, issues like self-esteem, achievement, mastery, independence, status, dominance, prestige. Only after esteem needs are met does the person seek self-actualization: realizing personal potential, self-fulfillment, looking for personal growth and peak experiences. Not all needs in an area must be met to seek the resolution of "higher" needs, but the person will likely feel some sense of mastery before moving on. Although selfless service is in the highest level, it has been found that individuals at lower levels will often provide unrewarded services to others in the right context.

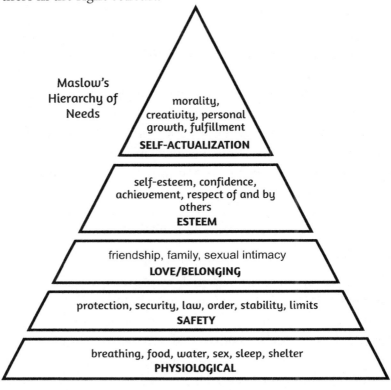

Fig 6.

It is important to recognize that your individual is unlikely to be operating at the same level as you. This may seem obvious, but often a clinician can see what they feel the individual should want and try to convince them of its usefulness. An example might be a new job, when the person is simply trying to create stability in their life after their separation. Discussion of a new job should come much later, if at all. Keep this prioritization scheme in your mind as you collaborate with the individual to develop their Individual Service Plan.

Develop the Goal

Once you have developed a list, and prioritized it, the next step is to state the goal in understandable terms. How do you know this should be a goal? What evidence do you have from the assessment? Can the goal be defined in behavioral terms?

When you and the person have agreed to focus on a particular area, the next step is to decide what they want to have happen. This is your long-term goal. Before you state this goal make sure it is something the individual can actually achieve and something that can be readily measured by both of you. Do remember that the person must desire the change or you both are wasting time; be sure to put things that are important to them high on the list, even if you can only do a small step toward accomplishing the goal.

Problem Solving

The following techniques are useful for collaborating with an individual to find solutions and make changes. It is a format typical to business and very useful in everyday life. The first two steps may be the most difficult part of the whole process.

- Define the difficulty. What specifically is the problem? The problem cannot be global or unclear and needs to be focused on the individual. If the problem is too large, it usually contains more than one problem and needs to be broken down into parts. The size of the problem is what often overwhelms the person and results in his/her giving up.
- Define the goal. What specifically is the goal? The goal cannot solve the problem if you don't know where you're headed. It needs to be realistic and attainable. Use the individual's words.

- Brainstorm for possible solutions. Do not censure any possible solution no matter how ridiculous it may sound; wild solutions can often be toned down and may trigger an idea for a more realistic solution.
- Evaluate the possible solutions for consent. If the individual dislikes it, you'll be unable to get commitment to action.
- Prioritize the solutions remaining. Pick at least the top three.
- Select one solution and put it into action. The best plan in the world is useless if no action is taken; it is essential to get the individual's commitment to follow through on the plan.
- Have a disaster (back-up) plan in place. This gives a feeling of confidence so the individual is more willing to take the risk of trying the #1 solution; if #1 doesn't work, maybe #2 will.
- Set a reasonable amount of time for re-evaluation and mark it on your calendar.
- Re-evaluate when the time comes.

Establish Objectives

Establishing short-term objectives is the next step. Identify one or two activities that can take place within a reasonable amount of time. Your individual moves closer to the goal each time one of these activities is accomplished. Now that you know where you are going, you need to determine how you are going to get there. There should be two objectives for each goal - begin small. Target dates should be set for each step. New objectives may be added to the plan to reflect the individual's progress or lack of progress. When the objectives have been met, the goal is achieved.

Points to Remember

- The goal must be stated or defined as a behavior that can be changed. It should be stated in terms easily understood by the individual.
- The objective must be measurable. Questions to ask are "How much change?" and "How do we know when the change has occurred?"
- The means or method used to attain the objectives must be reasonable and there must be a target date or time frame for each objective. The method should address what the individual will actually do, so it is essential to use active language. Use the dictionary or a taxonomy such as Bloom's for ideas (see Resources section).

Measuring Change

How do we measure change? Visible objective criteria are the most acceptable. Testing instruments, depending on their validity, are often considered the best methods of measurement but there are many changes they cannot measure. Third party observation is a valid measure of many behavioral changes. For instance: urinalysis is an example of visible objective criteria. A testing instrument cannot measure AA attendance. Third party observations may be solicited from the family or the employer. The clinician's own observations may be acceptable but there is a high potential for bias. The clinician's observations tend to be more acceptable if they are accompanied by observations of other staff, especially in the case of behavioral change.

While it's not always reliable, the individual's self-report should not be dismissed without due consideration. Self-report, while open to questions of validity and reliability, may be the only information available. Sometimes, taking the individual's word at face value develops into an important treatment strategy.

Use Your Creativity

Some creative ways to define, design and implement Individual Service Plans:

- Develop a list of usual problem areas using defining questions with a ranking scale (such as "agree-disagree). Have your individual rank their difficulties with various areas. Example: "My communication with my family needs improvement."
- Ask group members to brainstorm various problem areas, resulting goals, and suggest means to solutions, like books, activities, etc. Have everyone pick one that applies to them. Have them come up with means to solve it. Have each individual set time frames for themselves. Review each plan with the group, soliciting feedback and strategies for accountability.
- Develop "prizes" for people who have attained various treatment goals. These are best if acknowledged as a part of the group process.
- Create an "activity bank" defining various activities that individuals have used to achieve goals. These can be unique to your community, culture or area.
- Build a calendar for the individual with their deadlines stated for various tasks. Have them set rewards for themselves for reaching their goals.
- Have the individual do a drawing and/or a collage to represent 1) the problem, 2) the solution and 3) the means to achieve the solution.
- Develop forms and formats that allow individuals to keep track of their progress on various tasks. Share these in group on a regular basis.

· Review all plans for an active component. Have individuals be able to demonstrate to you and others that they have learned or mastered a solution through role plays, demonstrations, storytelling or physical evidence.

· If individuals seem stuck, use SNAP (see below) in a brainstorming mode to help with new ideas.

SNAP

One strategy that can be used to engage the individual in the treatment planning process is to do a SNAP analysis of the problem area. This consists of an analysis of the Strengths, Needs, Abilities and Preferences of the individual. You may wish to ask questions such as: "what is working right in this area?" or "how have you coped with the problem so far?" to elicit strengths. Needs should help clarify what is lacking, preferences will isolate a desired outcome. Drawing out abilities may take some coaxing on your part with your review of other life situations where the individual has succeeded – no matter how small – to pinpoint abilities that may have been overlooked by them.

Strengths	Needs	Abilities	Preferences
Creative	Uninterrupted sleep	Athletic	Same gender counselor
Honest	Stable employment	Good salesperson	Attend in evening
Intelligent	Medication evaluation	Good with kids	No written assignments
Good with money	Anger management	Public speaker	Counselor with history of addiction

Fig. 7

Documentation

As a clinician, you must be able to justify your decisions. Your diagnosis is based on the evidence in the assessment. If you indicate that therapeutic change has occurred you must show how and under what circumstances this happened. Progress notes must be connected to the objectives stated in the individual plan. If issues that are not listed keep coming up in counseling sessions, your Individual Service Plan needs reviewing. You must be able to defend everything that is written in the case record. If you keep current and clear with your documentation, no defense is necessary. If your documentation is not current, no defense is possible.

While paperwork is an important aspect of individual planning, there is much more involved than merely filling out required forms. Person centered planning is a global process that begins at intake and continues until discharge criteria are met or until services are discontinued. The document itself is a record of proposed individual services, written clearly and in easy to understand language that provides a guide for both the individual and clinician during the course of treatment. It also serves as a means of demonstrating compliance with licensing regulations and quality assurance. When linked to a formal review process, the Individual Service Plan becomes a major contribution to effective treatment.

The Individual Service Plan is a guide for both the person being served and the clinician. The implementation of the plan is the responsibility of the clinician but without individual agreement little progress will be made. Consideration must be given to the individual strengths and limitations of each individual. The plan must also be limited to goals that can be achieved during the treatment process.

Chapter Review

· What function does an Individual Service Plan play in a person's services and recovery process?

· What are the elements of an effective plan?

· Why is it essential to involve the patent and others, as appropriate, in the planning process?

Notes

[1] Maslow, Abraham, Motivation and Personality. (1954). New York: Harper & Brothers.

CHAPTER 7

Co-occurring Disorders

"Chaos is a friend of mine."

— Bob Dylan

Individuals who present for an assessment or treatment may be suffering from one or more disorders in addition to an addictive disease. The ultimate goal is holistic treatment, with concomitant conditions receiving coordinated care by suitable service providers when needed, possible and appropriate. The various domains that may be affected are biologic, psychological, social and spiritual. In the most straightforward case, a person may be addicted to drugs and also have a broken arm. Generally in the case of an acute condition such as a broken arm, the person will have been to urgent care or the hospital to have the bone set. Other than a probable follow-up to insure that the arm is being taken care of by visits to the doctor, and possible monitoring or investigation of pain medication, the counselor remains uninvolved with this condition.

In the case of a suspected but as yet undiagnosed co-occurring disorder, the counselor is bound by ethics and practice standards to investigate what intervention may be necessary. Possible co-occurring medical problems, such as untreated or unmanaged diabetes or high blood pressure, for example, are common in persons with alcoholism. Being familiar with signs and symptoms of these associated conditions, as well as resources for their treatment, is a requirement for good treatment professionals. This has been best practice for many years. A thorough physical is always a good idea for people in early recovery, even if the individual appears healthy. Particularly in the case of addicted adolescents, who look so much better so quickly, a physical examination is important to rule out anemia and other disorders that may sabotage recovery.

Definition

The term "co-occurring disorders" routinely refers to concurrent substance use and mental disorders in the current lexicon. Individuals said to have co-occurring disorders (sometimes abbreviated as COD) comprise one or more mental disorders as well as one or more disorders relating to the use of alcohol and/or other drugs. Other terms used to describe co-occurring disorders include "dual diagnosis," "dual disorders," "mentally ill chemically addicted" (MICA), "chemically addicted mentally ill" (CAMI), "mentally ill substance abusers" (MISA), "mentally ill chemically dependent"(MICD), "concurrent disorders," "coexisting disorders," "comorbid disorders," and "individuals with co-occurring psychiatric and substance symptomatology" (ICOPSS).

All disorders should be diagnosable using the current Diagnostic and Statistical Manual of Mental Disorders (DSM). In the case of co-occurring psychiatric disorders, the clinician may take different approaches, dependent on the type of disorder identified.

Differential Diagnosis

Differential diagnosis is defined as distinguishing between diseases of similar character by comparing their signs and symptoms. The ability of psychoactive substances to mimic nearly all the symptoms listed in the DSM 5 further complicates the task of differential diagnosis. Without additional information, it may be impossible to determine if the signs and symptoms reflect a naturally occurring mental illness or are the result of psychoactive substance use. The DSM 5 provides within many diagnostic categories the option of ruling out the diagnosis forcing the clinician to consider this diagnostic alternative.

Provided a good history has been taken, assessing the following issues can help clarify diagnosis:[1]

- Time of onset: If the psychiatric difficulties began or a diagnosis was made prior to the substance use, then it is likely that a psychiatric disorder exists. Using a timeline to clarify the appearance of signs and symptoms can assist in this determination.
- Patterns of substance use: A psychiatric disorder likely exists if the psychiatric symptoms persist during significant periods of abstinence from substance use (three months or longer). Diagnosis of a mental illness during a substantial period (one year or more) of abstinence from all drugs can provide support for a coexisting disorder.
- Consistency of symptoms: If the nature and magnitude of the symptoms and problems are qualitatively different or beyond what one would expect given the amount and type of substance used then a psychiatric disorder likely exists.
- Family history: Many psychiatric conditions, like substance use disorders, have a strong hereditary component. A

family history of mental illness can support the suspicion that a particular individual has a mental illness.

· Lack of response to treatment: individuals who suffer from both psychiatric and substance use disorders often have significant difficulty complying with traditional substance abuse treatment programs and relapse during or shortly after treatment.

· Individual's stated reason for substance use: Persons with a primary psychiatric diagnosis and secondary substance use disorders will often say that they "medicate symptoms" -- they drink to quiet auditory hallucinations, they use stimulants to ease depression, they use alcohol or another depressant to take the edge off anxiety or soothe a manic phase. Substance use will likely exacerbate psychotic conditions over time, but this does not mean that the psychiatric condition is substance induced.

If limited information prevents a firm diagnosis, the term "Provisional" may be used to indicate the lack of certainty. Although not part of the formal DSM-5 convention, many clinicians also use the term "Rule Out" or R/O (A term used in medicine, meaning to eliminate or exclude something from consideration) as a note prior to a diagnosis to indicate that not enough information exists to make the diagnosis, but it must be considered as an alternative.

The terms "provisional" and "rule out" can be particularly useful when trying to determine whether or not a client's symptoms stem from substance use or a psychiatric disorder. Onset and time(s) of abstinence may help sort out what diagnosis is most appropriate. If a particular client reported symptoms consistent with both major depression and alcohol dependence and had no significant periods of abstinence, this convention would alert others that the client's depressive symptoms may be caused by alcohol or may not resolve with abstinence and should continue to be assessed.

Treatment Approaches

The dually diagnosed individual has been treated historically with one of three general approaches:

- Sequential Treatment—treat one disorder first, then the other disorder.
- Parallel Treatment—treat both disorders simultaneously but in different settings.
- Integrated Treatment—treat both disorders simultaneously in the same setting.

Sequential Treatment

This method has been used historically, primarily because of the issues discussed earlier. The ability of substance use to mimic a number of psychiatric illnesses led to waiting until an individual had a length of abstinence from alcohol and other drugs before treating concomitant psychiatric disorders. The downside of this approach is that if the psychiatric disorder is serious, addiction recovery may be very difficult or impossible.

Parallel Treatment

Another method used for the treatment of psychiatric disorders and addiction has been used when it appeared that the psychiatric disorder – or the addictive disease – was interfering with the treatment of the other disorder. An example might be the mentally ill individual who used drugs and failed to take his psychiatric medication as needed, or the addicted person whose mood swings were so severe that he was unable to stay abstinent. This approach seemed more useful than sequential treatment, but since treatment generally takes place at different sites with different clinicians and little or no coordination, it can be less effectual than optimal.

Integrated Treatment

One of the goals of an integrated model for assessment, treatment and rehabilitation for mentally ill substance users is to provide a common language for mental health clinicians and professionals in the substance disorder field. Treatment is then matched to individuals with co-occurring or dual disorders. So far research has shown that several program features appear to be associated with effectiveness: assertive outreach (also known as assertive community treatment or ACT), case management, and a longitudinal, stage-wise, motivational approach to substance disorder treatment. Given the magnitude and severity of the problem of dual disorders, more controlled research on integrated treatment is needed.

Integrated treatment is preferred for this population as there is a high likelihood that individuals with psychiatric disorders will use, abuse, or become substance dependent. Use of substances relieves feelings of isolation, loneliness, and despair. With few alternative resources or the presence of cognitive impairments, the risk to turning to psychoactive substances is high.

Systems Changes

Recent decades have led to changes in our understanding of psychiatric diseases. There has been much research into biologically based brain disorders: mood disorders, post-traumatic stress disorder, anxiety and depression, rapid cycling disorders, obsessive compulsive disorder, impulse-control disorders, cognitive impairment disorders, attention deficit hyperactivity disorder, and anger-control disorders. We now know that these psychiatric diseases are 2-3 times more common in people who have substance-use disorders than in the general population. We are now more inclined to recognize that people with substance use disorders may have separate psychiatric disorders that require separate and distinct treatment. We now refer to these individuals as having co-occurring disorders[2].

Due to the perceived high incidence of co-occurring psychiatric disorders, many states have combined their alcohol/drug and mental health systems to better serve this population. This approach may not prove to be the best solution as it could artificially elevate the percentage of dually diagnosed individuals. As the ability to clearly and consistently define the various disorders improves – such as when the assessment is conducted and giving appropriate allowance for drug effects, both short and long term - the incidence of true co-occurring disorders may emerge. Watching for symptoms of a drug or alcohol masked psychiatric disorder is essential to insuring that relapse is prevented.

Standards of Care

Kenneth Minkoff, M.D was the chair of an expert panel that studied the Co-occurring Psychiatric & Substance Disorders in Managed Care Systems: Standards of Care, Practice Guidelines, Workforce Competencies and Training Curriculum. The panel posits that dually diagnosed individuals fall into one of the following categories:

Complicated Chemical Dependency - Psych-Low, Substance-High

Individuals with alcoholism or drug addiction who have significant psychiatric symptomatology and/or disability but who do not have serious and persistent mental illness. This category includes individuals who have both substance-induced psychiatric disorders and substance exacerbated psychiatric disorders. Psychiatric syndromes found in this category include:

· Anxiety/Panic Disorder

- Depression/Hypomania
- Psychosis/Confusion
- Post Traumatic Stress Disorder (PTSD) Symptoms
- Suicidality
- Violence
- Symptoms Secondary to Misuse/Abuse of Psychotropic Medication
- Personality Traits/Disorder

Substance Abusing Mentally Ill – Psych-High, Substance Low

Individuals with serious and persistent mental illness, which is complicated by substance abuse, whether or not the individual sees substances as a problem.

- Schizophrenia
- Major Affective Disorders with Psychosis
- PTSD that impairs work, social or personal functioning

Substance Dependent Mentally Ill – Psych-High, Substance-High

Individuals with serious and persistent mental illness, who also have alcoholism and/or drug addiction and who need treatment for addiction, for mental illness, or for both. This may include sober individuals who may benefit from psychiatric treatment in a setting which also provides sobriety support and twelve step programs.

Substance Abuse & Non Severe Psychopathology - Psych-Low, Substance-Low

Individuals who usually present in outpatient settings with various combinations of psychiatric symptoms and patterns of substance misuse and abuse, but not clear-cut substance dependence.

· Anxiety
· Depression
· Family Conflict

Recordkeeping Variables

In recordkeeping, the format of the case record depends on the requirements of the state as well as the scope of the program. Any co-occurring diagnosis as well as substance abuse should be clearly indicated when known. Co-ordination with medical providers is essential to good treatment, whether a co-occurring disorder or disease is identified or not. When psychiatric medications are indicated or prescribed, medical consultation is crucial and must be documented.

If sequential treatment is indicated, a comprehensive referral should be prepared for the mental health professional, including the individual's history, progress in treatment and their concerns. A follow up on the referral should be conducted to assure the individual has followed through and to link with the mental health provider in case additional information or assistance is needed.

Monitoring of any parallel treatment should be noted, as well as case staffing with a mental health professional who is managing the case. Any psychiatric medication being used by the individual should be discussed as part of treatment planning and knowledge of medication side effects demonstrated by the clinician. Since dually diagnosed individuals are high relapse risk, management of their mental illness and any required therapy and medications should be closely watched.

In integrated treatment, such as provided by a growing number of programs, case documentation will be defined by state regulation and program policy and procedure. No matter the format, the principles stated above are vital. The complications inherent in the case of the dually disordered individual make precise and current recordkeeping all the more important.

Parallels

Finally, persons with substance abuse disorder and mental illness have a number of things in common. Reviewing the parallels can give us new insights into both disorders and those who suffer from co-occurring disorders. We include here the 12 Parallels Between Chemical Dependency and Mental Illness from a colleague in Alaska, Michael Bricker, who treats individuals with addictive disease and mental illness[3]:

- Both are physiological diseases with strong genetic and hereditary components.
- Both are physical/mental/spiritual diseases which result in global affliction of the person.
- If left untreated, the course of both illnesses is progressive, chronic, incurable, and potentially fatal.
- Denial of the disease process and noncompliance with attempts to treat are cardinal symptoms of the disorder.
- Both diseases manifest loss of control in behavior, thought, and emotions. Both are often seen by self or others as a "moral issue."
- Both diseases afflict the whole family as well as all relational systems.

- Growing powerlessness and unmanageability lead to feelings of guilt, shame, depression, and despair.
- Both are diseases of vulnerability and isolation; the individual is exquisitely sensitive to psychosocial stressors.
- Both the primary symptoms of each disease AND loss of control in behavior/ thought/emotion are reversible with treatment.
- Recovery consists of: Stabilization of the acute disease; Rehabilitation of body, mind, and spirit; Launching upon an ongoing program of recovery.
- The risk of relapse in either disease is always high, and relapse in one disease will likely trigger a relapse in the other.
- The only hope for life-long recovery lies in working a recovery program(s): ONE DAY AT A TIME.

Chapter Review

- What are two types of dual diagnosis?

- Discuss different ways that individuals with dual diagnoses have been treated?

- Name three parallels between substance related disorder and mental illness.

Notes

[1] Adapted from Differential Diagnosis of Substance Use Disorders:
http://psycheval.com/substance%20_use_disorders.shtml. Gary L. Fischler & Associates, PA, Consulting and Forensic Psychologists, Minneapolis, Minnesota 55402.

[2] Co-occurring Substance Use and Mental Health Disorders in Adults: An Integrated Treatment Approach to Dual Diagnosis, Northeast ATTC, Pittsburg, PA. Download from ireta.org.

[3] Michael G Bricker, M.S., ICADC, LPC, Presented at the Alaska Annual School. Used with permission.

CHAPTER 8

Planning for Transition and Discharge

"If you don't know where you are going, you'll probably wind up somewhere else."

– Lawrence J. Peter

rom the beginning, both you and the person you are serving will want to have a clear understanding of what must occur before treatment ends. This means establishing, in conjunction with the individual, criteria for transition and discharge. You may find it useful to think of the transition plan as a document for the individual and the discharge summary as a document for the clinicians.

Transition

The process of transition planning should begin at admission. Transition is defined by The Commission on Accreditation of Rehabilitation Facilities (CARF) as "the process of moving from one level of care to another with the organization or to obtain services that are needed but are not available within the organization."[1]

Transition planning for post treatment helps the individual see that treatment goals are relevant to real life and that a workable maintenance plan will help to ensure continuing progress in recovery and prevent relapse. Direct and whole-hearted involvement can mean the difference between a plan that is followed and one that is ignored. Incorporating a person's strengths and preferences into the transition plan also helps to make the plan their own. When possible and practical, others, such as family, sobriety support, or concerned social service persons should be involved in the planning process. Encouraging the individual to make follow up appointments before leaving treatment or to visit places where he or she may want or need to go after discharge, especially from a residential setting, is highly desirable. This can help eliminate barriers to follow through.

A multidimensional view of the individual's needs should be considered when planning and a full array of supportive services should be available to transition planners. These would typically include consideration of services such as case management, child care, treatment of co-occurring issues of mental or physical health, realistic financial supports, and mutual support networking (such as twelve step programs). In some cases connections and communication with the legal system or child protection/family service agencies may be required.

Any transition period is particularly critical since it tends to place many pressures on the individual, the organization, and the community. Adequate preparation requires giving more than routine notice that the program is complete to the person served. It is necessary that there be early and active involvement in the transition planning process to ensure a solid foundation for recovery.

Developing the Transition Plan

A transition plan should be written as the individual is preparing to no longer be involved in intensive treatment and will be receiving only supportive counseling, even though the person has not been formally discharged and remains on the caseload of those receiving services from the treatment facility. In other words, the plan should be prepared for whenever a person's major active involvement in the treatment services changes or ends. Ideally, as the person reduces their involvement with the treatment agency and transitions to more time in the community, their plan becomes more complex and self-help focused. The Individual Service Plan leads to the transition plan. Many of the themes evident during treatment are naturally carried forward into the individual's life in recovery in the community.

Transition from treatment to community support or simply a step down in treatment frequency can be a time of increased pressure and intense adjustment for the individual. Creating a safety net in whatever form possible is essential. A thoughtfully crafted written transition plan can assist the individual to continue healthy habits and take advantage of resources to support and enhance their recovery. As with treatment planning, collaboration with the individual is essential.

When writing the plan, focus on the positive: have the individual visualize wellness for themselves. What does it look like, feel like, sound like? What are the needed steps to get there? Generally, staying sober is a key foundation for all the other goals. Use their "recovery capital"[2]– what are their strengths in the various life domains? If they have an interest and skills in computers, for example, how can that be used to their advantage? If they are an animal lover, what activities can be built into their life in recovery to include attention to this?

An effective transition plan should contain concrete, practical suggestions and strategies. "Go to the doctor" is open to interpretation. More useful is "Go to Dr. Jones for a follow up physical on May 10th at 2 p.m.", including Dr. Jones' location and contact information. Be sure to include simple rewards that can be easily obtained by the individual, such as watching a favorite movie after a difficult accomplishment or completing a task. If applying for a job is a challenge, create a reward for each interview or resume submission. The importance of written information cannot be over emphasized. Remember this is a brain disease with a built in "forgetter."

Encourage individuals to establish a routine that includes regular times and places for activities, particularly for activities that they enjoy. Help them to learn to practice behavior like mindful breathing and mindful walking and then write the practice on the plan as a regular activity. Include recovery maintenance tricks like deep breathing and responses to relapse triggers such as AA slogans, saying the Serenity Prayer or other quick "fixes" that work for the individual.

Relapse Prevention

The written transition plan includes referrals and a provision for forwarding information as appropriate. Relapse prevention plans should be an integral part of the transition plan. Terry Gorski writes "Preparation is often the key to succeeding in anything we pursue, including relapse prevention. We know that relapse is often part of recovery. Although not everyone relapses, those that do relapse can mitigate the destruction with a well-constructed and prepared relapse prevention plan. Relapse prevention planning can mean the difference between a short term relapse with minimal consequences, and losing everything in a long term bout with your substance abuse disorder."[3] It is vital to answer the question: if a relapse should occur, what actions should be taken? It is important to include the input and participation of the individual, the family, personnel and the referral source, as appropriate, in the transition plan. The plan should take into account the strengths, abilities, needs, and preferences (SNAP) of the individual, as well as their established and achieved preferences and expectations. Of course, the original transition plan should be kept by the person and a copy of the plan retained in the case record. Other persons who participate in the development of the transition plan could receive a copy of the plan, if appropriate and permitted.

Discharge

Discharge as defined by ASAM is the "point at which an individual's active involvement with a treatment service is terminated, and he or she is no longer carried on the service's records as patient."[4]

Discharge criteria must fit with the overall goals of the agency or facility providing treatment. A discharge from detox might include certain physical indicators of withdrawal stability while a discharge from intensive outpatient would likely show progress in a variety of psychosocial goals. It is also important to keep in mind that these criteria must be based on the person's individualized plans and goals and be in agreement with placement criteria, not the program structure (see Chapter 5).

If the individual is being treated in an outpatient setting, the ideal plan includes a number of contacts prior to formal discharge to set up community support. This is generally part of the transition process.

Writing the Discharge Summary

Discharge from a specific level of service may be either from that level to another or a complete discharge from treatment.

Discharge from one level of care to another within a continuum is commonly called "transfer or transition." This change should occur when the individual has achieved the treatment objectives that necessitated that level of care, for example reduction in craving symptoms. Use of the placement criteria will facilitate use of these clinical criteria, rather than time-related criteria such as program length.

The most common and most desirable reason for discharge is when the individual has achieved the Individual Service Plan goals or the majority of those goals. Although every attempt may be made to make an appropriate placement from initial assessment, treatment information may reveal a need to discharge or transfer the person. If the individual is unable or unwilling to work on appropriate treatment goals they may be transferred or discharged. In the case of an individual who is discharged due to lack of progress or simply drops out of treatment without warning, it is important to follow-up to assure that the individual is aware of their options. Relapse, while not an expected outcome, is prevalent and often the cause of treatment non-compliance. Providing alternatives to an individual who has relapsed affirms that the person is suffering from a disease, rather than being a "bad person" or "weak willed" and increases the likelihood that they will eventually seek recovery. Building a new life is not an easy thing to do.

As discussed above, when a person is close to discharge, three things should occur:

- Assist the individual in making contact with necessary agencies or services,
- Finalize the Transition Plan, and
- Provide the individual with a copy of the Transition Plan.

Once a person has been discharged, the counselor for each person should prepare a narrative discharge summary taking into account the individual's recent status and progress in treatment. This narrative includes the initial diagnosis, a description of the course of treatment, the individual's response to treatment and their condition at discharge, as well as the reasons for discharge. Recommendations and arrangements for further treatment, as appropriate, are documented. The dates of admission and discharge will also be included. The document or notation should be completed within a reasonable amount of time after discharge, no more than seven days.

In summary, discharge or transfer is a time of increased stress. An emphasis on planning and acknowledgment of this stress is helpful. Part of this acknowledgment consists of the identification of the patient's strengths and resources useful to ongoing recovery maintenance.

Chapter Review

· What are the elements of an effective transition plan?

· Why is it essential to involve the patent and others, as appropriate, in the planning process?

· Why should a discharge summary be prepared and what should it contain?

Notes

[1] 2014 CARF Behavioral Health Standards Manual July 2014 - June 2015

[2] White, W. & Kurtz, E. (2005). The Varieties of Recovery Experience. Chicago, IL: Great Lakes Addiction Technology Transfer Center

[3] Gorski, Terry "Early Intervention Planning in Relapse Prevention," http://www.friendsofrecoveryvt.org Accessed June 2008

[4] Mee-Lee D, Sulman GD, Fishman M, Gastfiend DR and Provence, Scott, eds. (2013) The ASAM Criteria, Third Edition, Chevy Chase MD: American Society of Addiction Medicine, Inc.

CHAPTER 9

Overview of Case Management

"There is no higher religion than human service. To work for the common good is the highest creed."

— *Woodrow Wilson*

Case management is defined as the administrative, clinical, and evaluative activities that bring the individual, treatment services, community agencies, and other resources together to focus on the issues and needs that were identified in the Individual Service Plan. Case management establishes a framework of action for the achievement of specified goals.

Another similar definition, developed for the Addiction Counseling Competencies Technical Assistance Publication sums up the various functions: Service coordination, which includes case management and client advocacy, establishes a framework of action for the client to achieve specified goals. It involves collaboration with the client and significant others, coordination of treatment and referral services, liaison activities with community resources and managed care systems, client advocacy, and ongoing evaluation of treatment progress and client needs.[1]

Models of Case Management

The long established social work model of case management is a broad based cradle-to-grave process. This model was developed for people who for one reason or another had needs that required ongoing support and advocacy, and included people with persistent and chronic mental illness or those who were developmentally disabled. Case management, in this context, generally means help with everyday needs. Often the work is quite intensive with one or more contacts per day - sometimes for a lengthy period of time. One case management model that is currently used with substance dependent individuals and mimics this service is the Assertive Community Treatment Model (ACT). See Fig 8.

Case management contains a wide variety of activities and intensities. As the addiction treatment field expanded from treatment only in the late 1960s to programs that included a variety of vocational and support services, the case management boundaries between other disciplines and ours began to blur.

As a result of the customary life problems brought on by substance related disorder, case management has become an integral part of the provision of the continuum of care. When we discuss case management for the people we serve it is a reference to the process of treatment, treatment support activities and follow up. Individuals in these settings are not necessarily chronically disadvantaged and working toward autonomy, but looking to regain stability in their lives. In general, the processes and specific activities cited in social work and mental health and substance abuse disorder treatment may overlap, or be the same, but the ultimate outcomes are likely to be different. Stabilization in social work and mental health means freedom from crisis – an impossible task unless an addicted person is abstinent and in recovery.

Chronically mentally ill individuals are unlikely to go for long periods of time without requiring services; recovering alcoholics and addicts are expected to do so and the nature of case management currently provided reflects these differences. Longitudinal research done in Illinois on individuals with substance related disorder treated in public facilities has shown that this expectation may be faulty. Of individuals who complete treatment between 25% and 35% of them are readmitted to treatment within one year; 50% may be readmitted within two to five years. In other words, up to 75 - 85% of the people we serve are readmitted to treatment. This means that acquainting the individuals we serve with good community supports is even more important than once thought.[2]

Record keeping is an essential component of case management and all the activities discussed here should be noted in the case record. Policies and procedures regarding case management activities must be carefully crafted and readily available to staff members.

Goals of Case Management

- Continuity of Care – At any time, the services provided to an individual are comprehensive, coordinated and continue over time, and are responsive to ongoing changes in the person's needs.
- Accessibility - Assist in overcoming the administrative barriers of multiple programs, each with its own eligibility criteria, regulations, policies and procedures.
- Accountability – Designation of a single point of responsibility for the overall effect of the system when multiple agencies are involved in meeting an individual's needs.
- Efficiency - Increasing the likelihood that individuals will receive the right services, in proper sequence and in a timely fashion. May or may not result in cost savings.[3]

Case Management Primary Functions

Knowing the functions and skills required for good case management is critical for today's clinician. A framework for case management activities and functions is supplied in the Addiction Counseling Competencies developed by the Addiction Technology Transfer Center Network (ATTCs), established by SAMHSA to transmit current information on treatment to providers in the field. Referral and service coordination are two of eight practice dimensions the ATTCs deem essential to the effective practice of addiction counseling. Activities considered part of those two dimensions include engagement; assessment; planning, goal-setting, and implementation; linking, monitoring, and advocacy; and disengagement.[4]

- Identification, Outreach and Engagement – Many case management programs attempt to enroll individuals not using customary services. They may work with, or be part of, a program such as a needle exchange, for example.
- Assessment – Determining an individual's current and potential strengths, weaknesses and needs. Generally this is done face to face but may be done by phone or electronically with proper safeguards.
- Planning – Developing a specific service plan for each individual .
- Goal Setting – Assisting the individual to set realistic and achievable short term and perhaps long term goals.
- Implementation – Maintain ongoing contact with the individual and others to ensure the plan is appropriate and working.
- Linkage – Referring or transferring individuals to all services in the formal and informal care-giving systems.

- Monitoring – Continuous evaluation of individual progress and assisting when necessary.
- Advocacy – Interceding on behalf of an individual to assure equity, both in the specific case and for any larger group or class to which the individual might belong.
- Disengagement – Working with the individual to create collaborative disengagement with appropriate transition planning and follow up.

Case Management Additional Functions

- Crisis Intervention – Short-term, brief, directed therapy as needed to intervene in a crisis that interferes with individual progress in achieving treatment goals and objectives.
- System Advocacy – In contrast to individual advocacy, a case manager often must confront entrenched administrative barriers to access services, but this advocacy may create conflict with the employee's own organization or among several organizations.
- Resource Development – The role of the case manager may be to take an active part in creative resource development.

Case Management Perspectives[5]

Broker/Generalist

This clinician helps to identify specific needs and assists an individual to find resources that can meet their needs. Generally this isn't a long term relationship and is typified by a short term association with a helper who supports the individual to find an appropriate treatment resource.

Strengths Perspective

Case management in this model is carried out by a team and is likely to be quite intensive, including help with tasks of daily living. Advocacy and contacts either at home or in community settings, such as drop in centers, is a primary component.

Assertive Community Treatment

The foremost two principles on which this model rests are (1) providing individuals support for asserting direct control over their search for resources, such as housing and employment, and (2) examining their own strengths and assets as the vehicle for resource acquisition.

Clinical/Rehabilitation

This model is the one most likely seen in small, community based organizations with behavioral health as the primary modality of treatment. Practitioners are trained in both therapy and case management activities and expected to provide services in both areas to their persons served.

Activities in Case Management				
Primary Activities	Broker Generalist	Strengths Perspective	Assertive Community Treatment	Clinical Rehabilitation
Conducts outreach and case finding	Not usually	Depends on agency mission & structure	Depends on agency mission & structure	Depends on agency mission & structure
Provides assessment and ongoing reassessment	Specific to immediate resource acquisition needs	Strengths-based, applicable to any of client life areas	Broad-based, part of a comprehensive (biopsychosocial) assessment	Broad-based, part of a comprehensive (biopsychosocial) assessment
Assists in goal planning	Generally brief, related to acquiring resources, possibly informal	Client-driven, teaches specific process on how to set goals and objectives, goals may include any of client life areas	Comprehensive, goals may include any of client life areas	Comprehensive, goals may include any of client life areas
Makes referral to needed resources	Case manager may initiate contact or have client make contact on own	As negotiated with client, may contact resource, accompany client, or client may contact on own	As needed, many resources integrated into broad package of case management services	As negotiated with client, may contact resource, accompany client, or client may contact on own

Primary Activities	Broker Generalist	Strengths Perspective	Assertive Community Treatment	Clinical Rehabilitation
Monitors referrals	Follow-up checks made	Close involvement in ongoing relationship between client and resource	Close involvement in ongoing relationship between client and resource	Close involvement in ongoing relationship between client and resource
Provides therapeutic services beyond resource acquisition, e.g., therapy, skills-teaching	Referral to other sources for these services if requested	Usually limited to responding to client questions about treatment issues, education about how to identify strengths and about self-help resources	Provides many services within unified package of treatment/case management services	Provision of therapeutic activities central to the model
Primary Activities	Broker Generalist	Strengths Perspective	Assertive Community Treatment	Clinical Rehabilitation
Helps develop informal support systems	No	Development of informal resources - neighbors, church, family - a key principle of the model	Through implementation of drop-in centers and shelters	Emphasis on family and self-help support through therapeutic activities
Responds to crisis	Responds to crises related to resource needs such as housing	Responds to crises related to both resource needs and mental health concerns; active in stabilization and then referral	Responds to crises related to both resource needs and mental health concerns; active in stabilization and then referral	Responds to crises related to both resource needs and mental health concerns; will stabilize crisis situation and provide further therapeutic intervention

Primary Activities	Broker Generalist	Strengths Perspective	Assertive Community Treatment	Clinical Rehabilitation
Engages in advocacy on behalf of individual client	Usually only at level of line staff	Assertive advocacy, will pursue multiple administrative levels within agency	Assertive advocacy, will pursue multiple administrative levels within agency	Assertive advocacy, will pursue multiple administrative levels within agency
Engages advocacy in support of resource development	Not usually	Usually in context of specific client needs	Either advocates for needed resources or may create resources as part of case management services	Usually in context of specific client needs
Provides direct services related to resource acquisition as part of case management, e.g., drop-in center, employment counseling	Referral to resources that provide direct services	Provides services crucial to preparing client for resource acquisition activities, e.g., role playing, accompanying client to interviews	Provides many direct services within unified package of treatment/case management	Provides services that are part of rehabilitation services plan; skill-teaching

Fig. 8.

Case Management Staff Positions

Broker Case Manager - Determines individual needs, develops Individual Service Plans, and/or refers individuals to agencies that will address identified needs. Often, these case managers monitor compliance with the Individual Service Plan and review and update the plans as necessary. Broker case managers often work with utilization review (UR) companies performing concurrent case reviews or transfer/discharge planning.

Program-Based Case Manager – The case manager is employed by a residential hospital unit, residential rehabilitation agency, or outpatient program providing case management as part of other responsibilities. Often, these case managers are employed as therapists in staff model treatment programs and perform only primary treatment duties.

Community Organizer Case Manager – The focus is helping the individual recover through community support and 'grass roots' movements (AA, NA, and Al-anon). Often, the case manager utilizes contacts within the 12 Step groups community to facilitate long-term recovery. Support can also be given to community group members by the case manager.

Counselor Case Manager – Here, the case manager is also the focal therapist, providing individual counseling, group therapy, didactic, and service brokering. In larger treatment agencies, these case managers may turn transition responsibilities over to social workers or outpatient counseling staff.

Full Service Case Manager – This case manager, as part of an interdisciplinary team, provides ongoing assessment, treatment, and follow-up. Few referrals are made to other agencies and most treatment services are provided by the team or the case manager. Historically, this type of case management best reflects the Minnesota Model of care utilized by treatment centers for close to 50 years.

Paraprofessional Case Manager – Trained volunteers or paraprofessionals, these case managers will help the individual as he/she becomes reintegrated into the community. The emphasis here is on informal and ongoing support. These case managers perform the role that was once filled by residential treatment program alumni associations.[6]

A Special Note About Referral

To properly implement a case management function, policies and procedures are required, and nowhere is this more important than in the referral process. Resources for various networks and referral options should be compiled and accessible in a central location, either electronic or physical. Information should be clear as well as guidelines for:

- Who to refer
- When to refer
- Where to refer
- How to make the referral

The primary goal of case management is to facilitate recovery for individuals and their families in our care; the process of referral may require knowledge levels from basic to quite sophisticated. When referring someone to another component in the same program, only specific program criteria are needed. Conversely, much skill and experience is needed to know when to refer a sexually abused individual to a therapist skilled in treating such issues. Successful referrals are not a "one size fits all" process.

In the Community

Another important aspect of this procedure is the development of community liaisons with appropriate resources. It is essential to always review the legal and ethical requirements or constraints placed on your action. Safeguards are recommended to ensure that appropriate consent and information protection procedures are implemented.

In summary, the term "case management" is used in a variety of settings and may mean different functions depending on the system in which it is used. In general, it refers to the functions and activities undertaken by a clinician or team of clinicians to support the recovery of the individual. Most of the tasks discussed in this chapter are carried out by counselors and other staff members in substance use disorder treatment programs.

Chapter Review

· How would you define case management?

· Explain how case management fits within the substance abuse disorder treatment system.

· The role of the case manager may be to take an active part in creative resource development. What could this include?

Notes

[1] Addiction Counseling Competencies: The Knowledge, Skills, and Attitudes of Professional Practice, Technical Assistance Publication (TAP) Series 21

[2] http://www.williamwhitepapers.com. Accessed July 15, 2014.

[3] Intagliata, J., Improving the Quality of Community Care of the Chronically Mentally Disabled: the Role of Case Management. Schizophrenia Bulletin, 1982, 8(4), 655-674.

[4] TAP 21: Addiction Counseling Competencies

[5] Comprehensive Case Management for Substance Abuse Treatment, Treatment Improvement Protocol (TIP) Series, No. 27, Center for Substance Abuse Treatment, Rockville (MD): Substance Abuse and Mental Health Services Administration (US); 1998, NCBI Bookshelf. A service of the National Library of Medicine, National Institutes of Health.

[6] Eiel, Christopher, M.A., LPC. Recovery Management Consultants, Lincoln, NE. Presentation, CARF Behavioral Health Winter Conference, Tucson, AZ 1995.

CHAPTER 10

Quality Assessment & Record Review

"A life spent making mistakes is not only more honorable, but more useful than a life spent doing nothing."

— *George Bernard Shaw*

The purpose of the quality assessment (QA) or quality improvement (QI) process is to continually monitor and evaluate the services provided by an organization. This process is undertaken to ensure that effective, efficient, high quality individual care is provided. Numerous areas of agency operations, such as risk management, staff credentialing, individual satisfaction and financial operations are reviewed in the QA process.

Scope

Depending upon the size and complexity of the organization, the staff member time devoted to this function might range from a few hours a month to full time for an entire department with many employees. Several tasks are performed to assist in fulfilling that purpose:

- Collecting, monitoring, documenting and maintaining sufficient data and interpretive information regarding clinical judgment to verify demonstrated competence for specific clinical privileges.
- Establishing and measuring staff member performance based upon objective job competencies and annual reviews. Assessing the performance of trainees is included here.
- Assuring that all clinicians are providing services in compliance with local, state, and federal regulatory agency guidelines.
- Assessing training needs of staff members and providing continuing education as needed.

For our examination of quality assessment, we will focus on the elements that reflect directly on the individual record. What follows is an abbreviated discussion on the elements of records review.

Process and Documentation

The QA Process and the documentation it generates are confidential. Quality assessment findings are documented so that the information may be used in a variety of ways. This information is often collated and presented to the appropriate supervisors. Various training or corrective actions can result. Depending on the information and its content, a Board of Directors or other leadership may review significant details to help with their decision making processes. Quality assessment information is used in documents such as an annual management report for the organization.

Records Review

This element of QA consists of the review and evaluation of aggregate information on case records to determine that they are:

- Organized – adequate in format and content
- Clear – effectively describe the condition and progress of the individual, and the treatment provided
- Complete – sufficiently inclusive (at all times) to facilitate continuity of care and communication between all those providing individual care services in the program
- Current – demonstrate timeliness to permit individual care reviews and other quality assessment improvement activities to be performed

In addition, a technique may include a review of standard practices relating to case records, including case records completion, procedures for maintaining confidentiality, forms, formats, filing, indexing, storage, availability, and recommendations of methods to ensure compliance with regulatory and accreditation bodies.

The QA process for record review can be conducted in a number of ways. All of the review processes listed below use a standardized review form that generates information on quality of care, utilization of resources, and conformance with key documentation requirements. These may differ slightly, but generally follow a similar format.

Outside Review

An outside reviewer may contract to provide this service. They would, of course, be subject to the same confidentiality laws as an employee. Confidentiality and privacy issues would be addressed as part of the service agreement. Any reports would be provided to the appropriate supervisor. Record reviews are often done as part of an audit or survey by a state authority or an accreditation body. This information, appropriately redacted - removing all individual identifying information - is generally included in the site visit report.

Case Records Committee Review

Another method of records review is a Case Records Committee (CRC) whose membership might include, for example: Director of Clinical Services; Residential Services Supervisor; Adult Outpatient Services Supervisor; Family Intervention Program Coordinator; Youth Supervisor; Youth Outpatient Services Supervisor; Administrative Assistant. Meetings could be scheduled monthly. The CRC would review a select sample of records and report on their findings. This information would be included in a QA report. The Executive Director might review the CRC meeting minutes, related documentation, and reports.

Peer Review

A peer review system uses clinical staff members to audit records prepared by their peers. This system has some advantages, including the in-service training that takes place during the process. Leadership of the review can rotate within the clinical staff members and depending on the organization size, may include only a portion of the clinical staff. It is not appropriate to allow an individual to review his or her own clinical documentation without supervision and feedback. An essential building block of a system using peer review is a clear standard with which to measure the various elements of the review. This can assist in conducting a non-biased evaluation of the record contents. On an individual basis, the records are returned to the clinician for correction. Corrective actions are tracked by the supervisor.

Elements of the Record Review

There are a number of elements commonly reviewed in the QA records review. We list some of the items below with some explanation to help understanding of what the terms mean.

The record should be completed promptly and all areas should be addressed. Blank lines or unsigned lines should not be present. Any non-applicable areas should be lined through or filled in with N/A. Unsigned documents should be filled in "refused" or whatever is appropriate. The assessment and other documents should be completed and available in the record within the time frame specified by policy and procedure.

Assessment

One element is the thoroughness of the assessment. Is it responsive to person's unique characteristics? The assessment should be individualized for each person served. It should address the person's culture, age, gender, sexual orientation, family history and situation, socioeconomic life, religion, spiritual orientation, etc. Using a boilerplate assessment narrative will not meet this intention – in other words, assessments where the same language is used to describe every individual. Individualized assessments should lead naturally to individualized narratives and Individual Service Plans.

Another element is the completeness of the assessment. Are all essential areas addressed? The clinician performing the assessment should note the presenting issue(s). What brought the individual to the treatment program? What is the first statement of difficulty the individual offers to the clinician? This is how the individual "introduces" themselves to the program.

After the assessment is completed, what are the expectations of the staff regarding the progress or responsiveness of the individual to the treatment process? Expectations should be clearly noted in assessment documentation. The clinician's expectation should be based on the information contained in the assessment. This could be looked upon as a prognosis – what is likely to happen to this person in the course of their treatment?

Another component reviewed is the individual's expectation of this treatment program. Is the individual actively objecting to treatment? Does the individual feel coerced into treatment? How ready is the individual to change? If willing to accept treatment, how strongly does the individual disagree with others' perception that he or she has a substance abuse disorder problem? Does the individual appear to be compliant only to avoid a negative consequence, or do they appear to be internally distressed in a self-motivated way about their alcohol/other drug use problems? How are these issues, if present, addressed by the clinical team and how are they documented?

The record should include a narrative assessment that interprets the assessment data. This narrative, or interpretive summary is not a repeat of the assessment. It is an effort on the part of the clinician to integrate, interpret, compare and contrast different aspects of the individual's life. The clinician synthesizes the information into a document. This document helps to introduce the individual to the reader, as well as postulate their response to treatment interventions, based on history. Writing a good summary is an art. Assessment summaries can vary in length from one paragraph to several pages. The format of the summary is unimportant, but a general expectation of the contents should be provided in the policy and procedure. The assessment should identify SNAP (strengths, needs, abilities and preferences) (see Chapter 6).

Historical Information

Incidents of previous alcohol or other drug and mental health services should be recorded. Treatment episodes should include dates (s), time, type of service and status at discharge. Records from all previous treatments should be requested after appropriate releases of information are signed. If the individual's case record shows previous treatments or hospitalizations, two items should be present in the record: 1) appropriate signed releases and, 2) copies of past treatment records, if enough time has elapsed. This information should be integrated into treatment planning.

Medical history and present medical status should also be described: allergies, illnesses, disabilities, needed medicines, etc. Current mental status or observation on emotional/behavioral functioning should be noted. This can be informal (observational and anecdotal) or formal (using an assessment instrument that is valid and reliable). A comprehensive social and alcohol/drug history should be present.

Individual Service Plan Goals and Objectives

Individual plan goals and objectives should be based on the assessment results and the goals expressed in the person's words. In the language of the individual, what goals do they want to achieve? These goals are developed with the help of the clinician, of course. Goals may be written verbatim in the Individual Service Plan, or paraphrased by the clinician, depending on organization policies and procedures. Objectives should be appropriate to the person's culture and age. Age and developmental issues must be taken into consideration when treatment objectives are formulated.

Look for objectives based on SNAP (strengths, needs, abilities and preferences). This is often overlooked because most clinicians are trained to formulate assessments and Individual Service Plans out of a "problem matrix." Newer treatment modalities operate from a rehabilitation model: the individual is viewed as the prime decision maker in the planning and treatment processes. This does not mean the clinician hands over his or her clinical powers to the individual; it means a clinician forms a therapeutic relationship with the person to help them cope with a chronic condition.

The plan is modified as needed. The individual plan is not a onetime effort. Look for update sheets, notations of plan review in the progress notes, or multiple Individual Service Plans. Updates can take place during one to one sessions, clinical staffing meetings regarding the individual, after group, etc. Updates may be discussed between the individual and the primary clinician or between the individual and the treatment team.

Services Provided

Actual services should be related to measurable objectives. Assigning the individual "group three times weekly to deal with substance related disorder" does not meet the intent of this indicator. A specific objective must be defined and agreed upon by the clinician and individual. An example might be: "Attend group 3 times weekly until <date> to learn ways to cope with relapse triggers, such as ..." The learning can be measured by a test or a conversation with the individual.

Objectives should be achievable. A clinician needs to be aware of the limitations, experiences and strengths of his or her patient before the clinician writes a treatment intervention. Do the progress notes address objective achievements? Are older objectives signed off and new ones assigned? Look for evidence of objective achievements.

Each objective should have a target date and a completion date (time limited). "Ongoing" is not acceptable. Utilization review (UR) personnel, as well as clinicians, need a treatment objective "road map" so they can approve continued stays or transfers to other levels of care. Individuals receiving services are encouraged by seeing completed objectives.

Note the frequency of treatment interventions. How many times does the person attend group therapy; watch didactic videos; read the "Big Book?" These should be individualized. One person may attend group five times weekly, while another may attend group twice weekly. Frequency of treatment interventions normally will be reflected in the Individual Service Plan, progress notes and discharge summaries.

Transition and Discharge

Transition Plans should be begun as early as possible and show progress in development as well as relationship to the ISP. A transition plan should include evidence that it was developed early in the treatment process. The plan should identify the person's need for another level of care as well as a current SNAP analysis. Collaboration should be clearly documented and a copy be retained in the record of individuals who have been discharged. Specific instructions/objectives and individualization should be evident. The fact that the person discharged received a copy of the plan upon discharge should be documented.

Discharge summaries should include information about the diagnosis, course of treatment, what goals were accomplished, and what referrals were made at discharge. It should also describe the services provided and the reasons for discharge.

Additional Items to Review

Consents to release confidential information should be complete, dated and signed. If various tests - such as for tuberculosis or other communicable diseases - are required, the case reviewer should look for these. A review should be conducted to check for follow up on such events as missed appointments or if discharged, a follow up on transition activities.

Use of Information

A form containing all the pertinent elements for the particular treatment setting should be consistently available for use in the QA process. Use of a standardized form to conduct a records review allows the reviewer and the supervisor to collect all the review information and make decisions on how treatment is or is not being documented. This information can highlight the clinician's areas of competence or spotlight areas where the entire organization could use improvement. One possible outcome is additional training for all or select staff members.

Chapter Review

• What are some of the uses for a records review?

• What are some of the ways and by whom reviews are done?

• Name five essential elements that are surveyed during a records review.

• What are the four guiding principles for good records?

Abbreviations & Symbols

A

AA or A.A.	Alcoholics Anonymous
AAP	Association of Alcoholism & Addictions Programs
ACA	Associated Counsel for the Accused
ACOA	Adult Children of Alcoholics
A/D	Alcohol/Drugs
ADATSA	Alcohol Drug Addiction Treatment Support Act
ADIS	Alcohol & Other Drug Information School
ALC	Alcohol
ALS	Administrative License Suspension
AMA	Against Medical Advice
AMT	Amount
ANS	Autonomic Nervous System
AOB	Alcohol on Breath
APA	American Psychiatric Association
APPT	Appointment
APR	April
ASA	Against Staff Advice
ASAP	As Soon As Possible
ASSESS	Assessment
ASSIST	Assist / Assistant
ATTY	Attorney
AUG	August

B

BAC	Blood Alcohol Concentration or Content
BAL	Blood Alcohol Level
BARBS	Barbiturates

| BO | Blackout or Brownout or both |
| BRO | Brother |

C

CA	Cocaine Anonymous
CARF	Commission on Accreditation of Rehabilitation Facilities
CAU	Caucasian
CC:	Copy to
CD	Chemical Dependency
CDP	Chemical Dependency Professional
CIG	Cigarette
CL	Client
CLR	Clear (DOL)
CNS	Central Nervous System
CO	County (DOL)
C/O	Closed out, Complaints of
CONT	Continued
CONV	Conviction (DOL)
COUNS	Counselor
CPS	Child Protective Services

C

CWS	Children's Welfare Services
CRT	Court (DOL)
CSI	Client Substance Abuse Index
CSO	Community Service Office
CT	Court

D

d	Day
D	Deferred (DOL), Days, Divorced
DAPR	DUI Assessment Profile Report
DBHR	Division of Behavioral Health & Recovery
D/C	Discharge
DD	Dual Diagnosis
DEC	December
DEPT	Department
DEP	Drug Education Program
DEF PROS	Deferred Prosecution (DOL)
DETOX	Detoxification
DI	Driver Improvement (DOL)
DIST	District
DMT	Hallucinogens, Indolealkyamines
DOB	Date of Birth
DOH	Department of Health
DOL	Department of Licensing
DOT	Director of Treatment, Department of Transportation
DOWNERS	Sedatives, alcohol, tranquilizers and narcotics
DP	Deferred Prosecution
DR	Driver Improvement (DOL), Doctor
DS	Dictation Status
DSHS	Department of Social and Health Services
DSM 5	Diagnostic and Statistical Manual of Mental Disorders
DSP	Disposition (DOL)
DT	Delirium Tremens
DTD	Date or Dated
DUI	Driving under the influence of intoxicants
DWI	Driving while intoxicated

DWLS	Driving while license suspended
DWLR	Driving while license revoked
Dx	Diagnosis

E

EADEP	Extended Alcohol Drug Education Program
EAP	Employee Assistance Program
EAPA	Employee Assistance Professionals Association
ECU	Extended Care Unit
E.G.	Exempli gratia (for example)
ELIG	Eligible (DOL)
ENDR	Endorsement (DOL)
Etc.	Et cetera (a number of unspecified persons or things)
ETOH	Alcohol
EVAL	Evaluation
EXP	Expiration (DOL)

F

FAE	Fetal Alcohol Effects
FAM	Family
FAS	Fetal Alcohol Syndrome
FDA	Food and Drug Administration
FEB	February
FM	From
FR	Financial Responsibility (DOL)
FREQ	Frequency
FS	Final Status
FST	Field Sobriety Test
FTA	Failure to Appear (DOL)
FTC	Federal Trade Commission
FTP	Family Treatment Program

FIU	Follow-up
FWD	Forward
FYI	For your information

G

GA	Gamblers Anonymous
GAIN	Global Assessment of Individual Needs
GAF	Global Assessment of Functioning
GAU	General Assistance Unemployable
GM or gm	Gram
GED	General Education Degree

H

HASH	Hashish
HBD	Had been drinking
HP	Higher Power
H&P	History and Physical
H&R	Hit and Run
Hx	History
HTO	Habitual Traffic Offender

I

I/D	Identification Card (DOL)
ID or I.D.	Identification
IHS	Indian Health Services
ILL	Illegal (DOL), illness
IM	Intramuscular
IND	Individual
INFO	Information
INS	Insurance
INTOX	Intoxicated

IOP	Intensive Outpatient
IOPTX	Intensive Outpatient Treatment
IPTX	Intensive Inpatient Treatment
IS	Information School
ISS	Issue (DOL)
ITA	Involuntary Treatment Act
IV	Intravenous

J

J	Jail (DOL)
JAN	January
JCAHO	Joint Commission on Accreditation of Health Care Organizations
JOINT	Marijuana Cigarette
JR	Judicial Review
JUL	July
JUN	June
JUV	Juvenile (DOL)

L

LCB	Liquor Control Board
LIC	License
LSD	Lysergic Acid Diethylamide
LTR	Letter

M

M	Married
MAL.MIS.	Malicious Mischief
MAST	Michigan Alcoholism Screening Test
MAR	March

MBD	Minimal Brain Dysfunction
M/C	Motorcycle (DOL)
MESC	Mescaline
MG, mg	Milligram
MIC	Minor in Consumption
MIN	Minute
MIP	Minor in Possession
MISC	Miscellaneous
MMPI	Minnesota Multiphasic Personality Inventory
MO	Month
MPH	Miles per hour
MTH	Month
MOS	Month, Months
MUN	Municipal
MJ	Marijuana

N

NA	Narcotics Anonymous
N/A	Not applicable, No Account
N/A	No Action (DOL)
N/C	No Charge
NIDA	National Institute on Drug Abuse
NO	No Status Sent
NOV	November
NSP	No Significant Problem

O

O	Open
OBJ	Objective
OCT	October
OD	Overdose
ODL	Occupational Drivers License

OL	Operating License
OP	Outpatient
OPTX	Outpatient Treatment
OTC	Over the counter drugs

P

P	Page, After
PA	Public Assistance
PC or P.C.	Physical Control
PD	Public Defender
PDA	Public Defender Association
PDR	Physician's Desk Reference
PEI	Personal Experience Inventory
PEND	Pending (DOL)
PMT	Payment
P.O. or PO	Probation Officer
PROB	Probation (DOL)
POT	Marijuana
PIEF	Paid in Full
PP	Pages
PSE	Pre-Sentence Evaluation
PTE	Pre-Trial Evaluation
Px	Past History

Q

q	Every
QTR	Quarter

R

RCW	Revised Code of Washington

RE:	Reference made to
REDS	Barbiturates, secobarbital
REG	Regulation
REIN	Reinstatement (DOL)
REL	Release (DOL)
REM	Rapid Eye Movement
REV	Revocation (DOL)
R/O	Rule Out
RPT	Report, Reported
Rx	Prescription

S

S	Single
SASSI	Substance Abuse Subtle Screening Inventory
SEP	September
SO	Significant Other
SOAP	Subjective, Objective, Assessment, Plan
SPI	Significant Problem 1 (DOL)
SP2	Significant Problem 2 (DOL)
SR	Safety Responsibility (DOL)
SR22	Financial Responsibility
SS# or SSN	Social Security Account Number
STAT	Immediately
STP	Dimethoxymethylamphetamine hallucinogens Phenylethylamines
SUP	Superior (DOL)
SURR	Surrendered (DOL)
SURV	Surveillance (DOL)
SUS	Suspended
SUSP	Suspension (DOL)

T

T/C	Telephone Call
TB	Tuberculosis
THC	Tetrahydrocannabinal or Marijuana
TIA	Transient Ischemic Attack
TRAING	Training
Tx	Treatment

999U

UA	Urinalysis
UPPERS	Stimulants, Cocaine and Psychedelies

V

VA	Veterans Administration
VIOL	Violation (DOL)
VOL	Volume

W

W	Widowed
W/ or w/	With
W/in	Within
W/out	Without
WA	Washington
WAC	Washington Administrative Code
WASAM	Washington State Alcohol Monitoring System
WDP	Weekday Program
W/In	Within
WGT	Weight
WK	Week
WNP	Weeknight Program
W/O	Without

WSAIOP	Washington State Association of Independent Outpatient Programs
WSADC	Washington State Alcohol & Drug Clearinghouse
WT	Weight

X Y Z

X or x	Times
Y or y	Deferred Prosecution (DOL)
YR	Year
YSA	Youth Substance Abuse

Common Symbols

&	And
♂	Male
♀	Female
@	At
X	Times, By
%	Percent
#	Number or Pound
+	Plus, Add or Excess of
—	Subtract or Deficiency of
<	From, Less Than
>	Where, More Than
↑	Increase
↓	Decrease

1°	First Degree
2°	Second Degree
3°	Third Degree
1:1 OR 1 TO 1	One-to-One Counseling Session
=	Equals
∴	Therefore
C̄ or C̲	With
S̄	Without

Resources

Substance Abuse and Mental Health Services Administration

The Substance Abuse and Mental Health Services Administration (SAMHSA) is the agency within the U.S. Department of Health and Human Services that leads public health efforts to advance the behavioral health of the nation. SAMHSA's mission is to reduce the impact of substance abuse and mental illness on America's communities.

Their site contains a wealth of information regarding alcohol, drugs and treatment. Most of the publications are downloadable.

Examples:

- The Confidentiality of Alcohol and Drug Abuse Patient Records Regulation
- HIPAA Privacy Rule: Implications for Alcohol and Substance Abuse Programs (2004).

http://store.samhsa.gov/home

Alcohol & Drug Abuse Institute – University of Washington

The ADAI clearinghouse is a resource center for Washington State residents, with both print and online resources about drugs and alcohol.

http://adaiclearinghouse.org/

CIWA

The Clinical Institute Withdrawal Assessment of Alcohol Scale, Revised (CIWA-Ar) is a tool to assess withdrawal risk and can be downloaded from:

http://ireta.org/sites/ireta.sitesquad.net/files/CIWA-Ar.pdf

Bloom's Taxonomy and Revisions

There is more than one type of learning. A committee of colleges, led by Benjamin Bloom, identified three domains of educational activities:

- Cognitive: mental skills (Knowledge)
- Affective: growth in feelings or emotional areas (Attitude)
- Psychomotor: manual or physical skills (Skills)

Since the work was produced by higher education, the words tend to be a bit more complicated than we normally use. Domains can be thought of as categories. Trainers often refer to these three domains as KSA (Knowledge, Skills, and Attitude). This taxonomy of learning behaviors can be thought of as "the goals of the training process." That is, after the training session, the learner should have acquired new skills, knowledge, and/or attitudes.

http://www.nwlink.com/~donclark/hrd/bloom.html

Index

A

C

D

Documenting Services and
   Progress, 7
DSM-5, 56, 65, 66, 84
Dual disorder, 82
Dually diagnosed, 85, 87, 90

E

Electronic Medical Record, ii
EMR. *See* Electronic Medical
   Record

F

First Visit, 5

H

HIPAA, 26, 139
History and physical, 4

I

Initial Contact, 2
Integrated treatment, 86
Intervention, 4, 61, 100, 105,
   118

L

Late entry, 23
Literacy, 39

M

Medical necessity, 68
Medication, 19, 77, 88
Medicines, 68
Minors, 35

O

Objectives, 74, 121, 122

P

Parallel treatment, 85
Patient Placement Criteria,
   53, 54
Peer review, 118
Primary Record Elements of
   the Service Process, 6
Privacy, 25, 26, 139
Progress Notes, 16, 17, 18,
   19, 20, 21
Progress Notes Formats, 17

Q

Quality Assessment, 115
Quality improvement, ii, 115

R

Rapport, 38, 41
Recommendation, 49

ABOUT THE AUTHORS

Sherry Kimbrough is an experienced program & accreditation consultant, program developer, counselor and educator. She holds an M.S. in Psychology from Columbia Pacific University, Addiction Studies credentials from Seattle University and was first formally qualified as a Chemical Dependency Counselor in 1977. Sherry has taught chemical dependency courses at several colleges in Washington State and retired as an international surveyor for CARF International – the Commission on Accreditation of Rehabilitation Facilities in 2014 after 22 years. Loving to be the center of attention made her a natural to teach. She has direct experience as an Executive Director, Clinical Supervisor and Program Manager in both residential and outpatient chemical dependency treatment agencies. Since 1990, Sherry has developed and presented hundreds of hours of continuing education and cross disciplinary training in a variety of venues nationwide.

Landon Kimbrough has developed and implemented program evaluation systems for treatment providers in the United States. He is a recognized expert in technical assistance in designing and implementing corrective action plans and writing policies and procedures to assist chemical dependency agencies in maintaining certification. Landon successfully combines his many years of business experience and his position as former director of a hospital-based intensive residential treatment provider, developing an integrated clinical documentation system. He holds a Masters of Ministry in Religious Education from Seattle University.

CPSIA information can be obtained at www.ICGtesting.com
Printed in the USA
LVOW04s0721151214

418756LV00016B/354/P